Preface

This book is intended to be read by clinicians and trainees in general practice and internal medicine and to be useful in a practical and immediate fashion. Hypertension is a major, common medical problem, and one of the most common chronic diseases in the urban world. During the past decade, the management of hypertension has become a highly individualized process. Identification of patient subsets and a working knowledge of how to manage these patients therapeutically has become a necessity for the clinician working both in and outside of the hospital setting. Therapeutics has become much more complex in recent years, with not only the introduction of numerous new drugs, but new classes of drugs and new combination products as well. Physicians, therefore, want and need to use the available regimens to their best advantage.

This book has been organized into several sections that include descriptions of patient types and categories, the epidemiology and aetiology of hypertension, information on clinical trials and outcomes, diagnostic assessment of the patient and treatment of hypertension. As all the authors have expertise in clinical pharmacology, there is a significant focus on therapeutics and a detailed discussion of the various classes of antihypertensive agents. The treatment sections include discussions of the efficacy and adverse event profiles of various antihypertensive drug classes, as well as the special benefits and compelling reasons to use a particular antihypertensive drug for difficult-to-treat patients and those who have comorbidities that greatly influence drug selection.

Finally, a great deal of attention has been paid to an appendix of antihypertensive drugs and an appendix of useful addresses and websites, which will serve as a guide for the practicing doctor for the years to come. It is greatly hoped that the information provided in this book will be translated into better care of millions of hypertensive patients that ultimately will lead to achieving the important goal of reducing cardiovascular morbidity and mortality.

William B White MD, FACP
Farmington, Connecticut, USA
2003

Abbreviations

ABPM	ambulatory blood pressure monitoring
ACE	angiotensin-converting enzyme
ACEI	angiotensin-converting enzyme inhibitor
AT	angiotensin receptor subtype
BHS	British Hypertension Society
BP	blood pressure
CCB	calcium channel blocker
CHD	coronary heart disease
CI	confidence interval
COX-2	cyclo-oxygenase-2
CV	cardiovascular
CVD	cardiovascular disease
DBP	diastolic blood pressure
ET	endothelin
GITS	gastrointestinal therapeutic system
HDL	high-density lipoprotein
ISH	isolated systolic hypertension
JNC	Joint National Committee
LDL	low-density lipoprotein
LV	left ventricular
MI	myocardial infarction
NEP	neutral endopeptidase
NSAID	non-steroidal anti-inflammatory drug
PVD	peripheral vascular disease
RAAS	renin–angiotensin–aldosterone system
RR	relative risk

Introduction

Cardiovascular disease (CVD) is the second leading cause of mortality worldwide (Figure 1) and has been predicted to become the leading cause during the course of the next 20 years. Hypertension is a well-established risk factor for all forms of CVD (Figure 2). In the industrialized world, hypertension constitutes a considerable problem, because up to 20% of individuals may be considered to be hypertensive according to current definitions. However, even this figure may be misleading in that about 50% of individuals aged between 65 and 74 years have hypertension and among older patients the prevalence is even higher. Given the demographic changes which are predicted to occur in the next 50 years, it is clear that hypertension will assume even greater importance in the future (Figure 3). Since it is well recognized that hypertension is one of the major risk factors for cardiovascular (CV) mortality and morbidity, there are obvious and substantial future cost implications for healthcare systems.

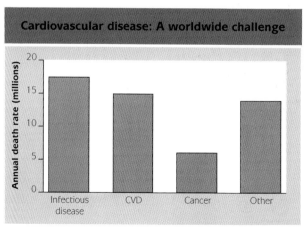

Figure 1. Leading causes of worldwide mortality.

The benefits of the effective treatment of hypertension have been well established in patients up to the age of 80 years and probably beyond. These benefits are mainly due to a reduction in the incidence of strokes, coronary events and heart failure: these morbidities are particularly important because they result in the loss of physical and mental capacity, especially in the elderly. The reductions in mortality are less clear-cut, but the overall protection against CV events in association with sustained reductions in blood pressure certainly indicates that treatment should be initiated in all eligible patients.

Thus, there is substantial and clinically meaningful evidence of benefit associated with clinical trials in patients with hypertension. However, the evidence from routine clinical practice throughout the world suggests that many patients remain undiagnosed and those who are diagnosed do not have their blood pressure adequately controlled despite the availability of a wide range of efficacious antihypertensive drugs.[1-3] In the late 1990s, less than 30% of patients with hypertension were normalized on drug therapy; this number is even lower for patients with diabetes,

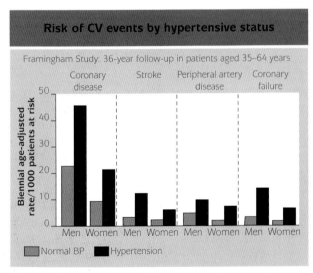

Figure 2. Hypertension as a risk factor for cardiovascular disease.

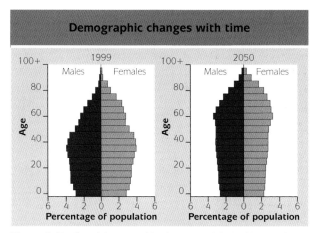

Figure 3. Predicted demographic changes and the incidence of hypertension.

renal insufficiency and coronary disease, where the goals of therapy are 140/90 mmHg. Statistics for the diagnosis, treatment and control of hypertensive patients in England and Wales are shown in Figure 4. Although there has been an improvement over a 4-year period, control rates remain low, particularly when focusing upon the more stringent blood pressure (BP) targets defined in recent guidelines for treatment.[3]

There is a further potential problem associated with hypertension management in that, even where treatment is seemingly effective in restoring "normal" blood pressure, it has not been shown to reduce the CV risk in the treated hypertensive patient to the level of risk seen in normotensive subjects, despite the attainment of an equivalent blood pressure (Figure 5).[4] Whilst sub-optimal blood pressure control or inadequate duration of treatment may contribute to this continuing excess risk, failure to adequately assess and control other concomitant CV risk factors is another pivotally important factor. Successful hypertension management therefore involves more than simply controlling blood pressure, and in order to maximize the benefit, all CV risk factors in an individual patient must be addressed for that patient to obtain the maximum treatment benefit.

The principal aim of this rapid reference text is to provide a summary of the information currently available on hypertension management and the selection of appropriate drug therapy.

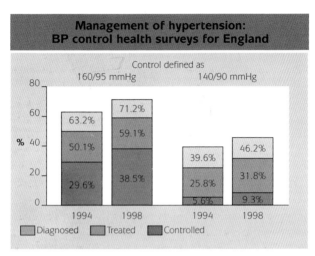

Figure 4. Health surveys for England and Wales: diagnosis, treatment and control of hypertension.

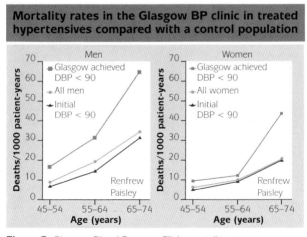

Figure 5. Glasgow Blood Pressure Clinic mortality rates: comparison of control populations with treated hypertensives. Data taken from reference 4.

Definitions: Epidemiology, Natural History and Prognosis

As blood pressure rises, it is associated with various adverse CV events. The relationship between blood pressure level and the risk of a CV event is a continuous one, and thus there can be no arbitrary dividing line between a blood pressure that is devoid of CV risk and a blood pressure that represents "significant" CV risk (Figures 6 and 7).[5] Considering that there is an interaction between blood pressure and other CV risk factors, and also ethnic and genetic differences, the prognostic significance of any given blood pressure reading will vary between different patients. Thus, in many respects the definition of "normal" blood pressure and hypertension are arbitrary.

Hypertension can be sub-classified into seven categories: essential hypertension, isolated systolic hypertension, pseudohypertension, white coat hypertension, secondary hypertension, accelerated hypertension and malignant hypertension.

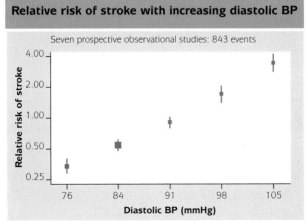

Relative risk of stroke with increasing diastolic BP

Figure 6. Diastolic blood pressure and the risk of stroke. Data from reference 5.

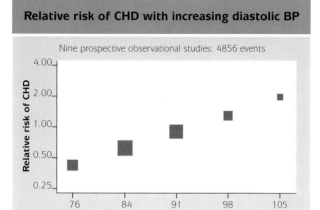

Figure 7. Diastolic blood pressure and the risk of coronary heart disease. Data from reference 5.

Essential hypertension

Essential hypertension is the most common form of elevated blood pressure and may be defined as an elevation of arterial pressure that results from the inappropriate regulation of normal homeostatic control mechanisms in the absence of a detectable cause. A number of different national and international organizations have promulgated guidelines on hypertension management and the definition of hypertension. The major guidelines are broadly similar and categorize levels of blood pressure according to severity. The definitions of blood pressure normality and grades of hypertension defined by the Joint National Committee on Detection, Evaluation and Treatment of High Blood Pressure (JNC VI) guidelines from the United States, along with those defined by the WHO-ISH guidelines of 1999, are shown in Table 1.[6,7] It is apparent that these definitions are broadly similar and both acknowledge that hypertension should be classified not only on the basis of arterial pressure, but also by overall CV risk. Accordingly, treatment should be based upon a stratification which takes account not only of the level of the blood pressure, but also of the other CV risk factors.

Definitions and classification of blood pressure levels

	1999 WHO/ISH guidelines			JNC VI guidelines		
Category	Systolic (mmHg)	Diastolic		Category	Systolic (mmHg)	Diastolic
Optimal	<120	<80		Optimal	<120 and <80	
Normal	<130	<85		Normal	<130 and <85	
High–Normal	130–139	85–89		High–Normal	130–139 or 85–89	
Grade 1 Hypertension (mild)	140–159	90–99		Hypertension Stage 1	140–159 or 90–99	
Subgroup: borderline	140–149	90–94		Hypertension Stage 2	150–179 or 100–109	
Grade 2 Hypertension (moderate)	150–179	100–109		Hypertension Stage 3	≥ 180 or 110	
Grade 3 Hypertension (severe)	≥ 180	≥ 110				
Isolated systolic hypertension	<140	<90		Isolated systolic hypertension	<140 and <90	
Subgroup: borderline	140–159	<90				

For both guidelines when systolic and diastolic blood pressures fall into different categories, the higher category should apply.

Table 1. Definitions and classification of blood pressure levels.

Isolated systolic hypertension

In industrialized societies, systolic blood pressure continues to rise with age whilst diastolic blood pressure tends to plateau around the age of 60 years and declines somewhat thereafter (Figure 8). This blood pressure pattern is associated with the loss of distensibility and elasticity in the large capacitance arteries, and is considered to be a reflection of relatively widespread arteriosclerosis. In this situation, systolic pressure is higher than normal whilst diastolic pressure falls within conventionally normal limits, resulting in the definition of isolated systolic hypertension (Table 1).

Pseudohypertension

In rare instances, blood pressures recorded by conventional cuff sphygmomanometry are elevated but do not reflect the true blood pressure as measured by intra-arterial monitoring. This is usually associated with relatively incompressible peripheral vessels caused by calcification of the arterial media and may occur in the absence of hypertensive end organ damage.

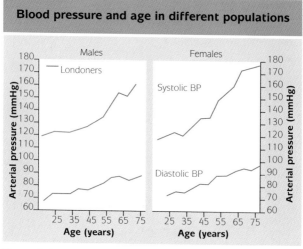

Figure 8. Blood pressure changes with increasing age in industrialized society.

White coat hypertension

Some patients exhibit elevated blood pressures when measurements are made in the clinic or office environment. In contrast, when blood pressure is assessed away from the clinical environment, usually by ambulatory recordings, pressures are considered to fall within the normal range (Figure 9). Such patients may have persistently elevated blood pressure when measured in the clinical environment, but little or no evidence of end organ damage. It was originally thought that this disorder was relatively benign, but it is becoming increasingly apparent that the CV risk in these patients may be intermediate between normal and sustained hypertension and that, in the long term, there may be a significant increase in risk. Additionally, of great importance is the value of ambulatory BP that is chosen to define white coat hypertension. In the PIUMA database in Italy, as well as the Ohasama population in Japan, patients whose ambulatory systolic BP is less than 130 mmHg, despite having hypertensive office BP readings, do not have excess risk of vascular events compared to normal, healthy age-matched subjects.[8,9]

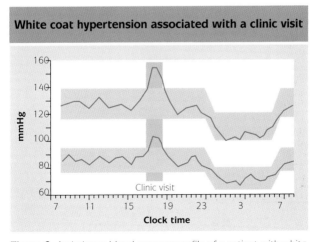

Figure 9. Ambulatory blood pressure profile of a patient with white coat hypertension.

Secondary hypertension

Secondary hypertension is usually defined as persistent hypertension which can be attributed to a definable underlying disorder (see section on clinical investigations).

Accelerated hypertension

Accelerated hypertension is the terminology applied in severe hypertension, with blood pressure around 200/120 mmHg and above, when significant target organ damage is present, usually in association with advancing renal insufficiency and fundoscopic haemorrhages, but in the absence of papillocdema or a medical emergency.

Malignant hypertension

Malignant hypertension may be defined as severe hypertension in association with one or more of the following:

1. Papilloedema
2. Pulmonary oedema
3. Neurological findings (hypertensive encephalopathy)
4. Hypertension-induced angina

It therefore seems to be the same as a hypertensive emergency – malignant hypertension has been classically defined as associated with fibrinoid necrosis of the arterioles and small arteries.

Epidemiology

On the basis of current evidence, it is reasonable to suggest that arterial hypertension is the consequence of the interaction between genetics and the environment (Figure 10). Inheritance makes an individual more susceptible to developing hypertension, while environmental factors help to accelerate the increase in blood pressure and the subsequent CV damage.

Whilst acknowledging that hypertension is almost certainly a polygenic disorder, its severity is often determined by other factors; increasing age and ethnicity are the two major factors in practice which determine the prevalence of hypertension in a given community.

Age

The distribution of blood pressure within most populations is essentially unimodal and normally distributed, with slight skewing at the upper end of the distribution (Figure 11). In

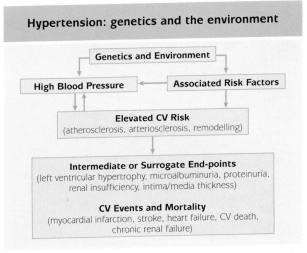

Hypertension: genetics and the environment

Genetics and Environment

High Blood Pressure ← Associated Risk Factors

Elevated CV Risk
(atherosclerosis, arteriosclerosis, remodelling)

Intermediate or Surrogate End-points
(left ventricular hypertrophy, microalbuminuria, proteinuria, renal insufficiency, intima/media thickness)

CV Events and Mortality
(myocardial infarction, stroke, heart failure, CV death, chronic renal failure)

Figure 10. Hypertension: the interaction between genetics and the environment.

such populations, the prevalence of hypertension increases with age. The age-related increase in systolic pressure continues until late in life, whereas diastolic pressure tends to plateau around the age of 60 years and thereafter may even fall slightly (Figure 8), resulting in an increased incidence of isolated systolic hypertension (ISH). However, this is largely associated with Westernized or industrialized populations and is not observed in more primitive societies (Figure 12). The increased incidence of hypertension in the elderly, in part, reflects the increasing prevalence of factors which contribute to the development of hypertension and atherosclerotic vascular disease, particularly obesity and reduced physical activity, which themselves increase in prevalence with increasing age. Basically, however, the age-related and progressive reduction in vascular compliance (or elasticity) is directly associated with an increase in peripheral vascular resistance and an increase in blood pressure.

Thus, ISH is a particular feature of the elderly hypertensive patient. It is usually attributed to the loss of compliance (elasticity) in the major blood vessels and is defined as a systolic

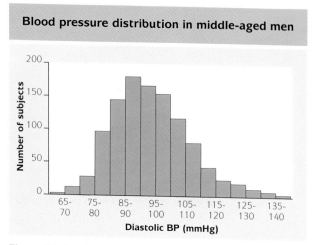

Figure 11. Distribution of diastolic blood pressure in a population.

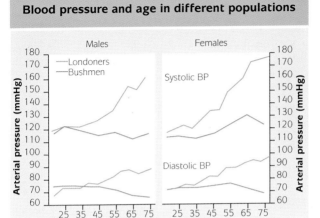

Blood pressure and age in different populations

Figure 12. Blood pressure changes with increasing age in a non-industrialized and industralized society.

blood pressure of 160 mmHg or above, in association with a diastolic pressure of 90 mmHg or less. The prevalence of ISH is about 15–20%, but it is clearly associated with increasing age and may involve the majority of the population aged over 80 years.

From the Framingham database, it was established that the mortality from all causes was doubled in those men aged 55–74 years with ISH, compared with age-matched normotensive individuals (Figure 13).[10] Correspondingly, CV death is almost two-fold more frequent in men with ISH and almost five times more frequent in women with ISH, compared to normotensive individuals. Finally, the risk of stroke is increased by two- to four-fold if ISH is present and this risk increases as the actual level of systolic blood pressure increases in relation to diastolic pressure, i.e. in association with a progressive increase in pulse pressure. Some studies have suggested that, of all the measures of hypertension, pulse pressure is the most important determinant of CV risk.[11,12] However, as pulse pressure is

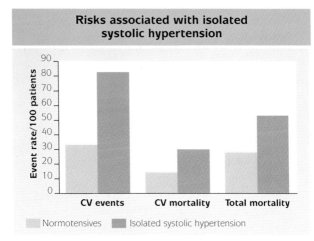

Figure 13. CV events in patients with normotension and isolated systolic hypertension. Data from reference 10.

directly derived from the difference between systolic and diastolic pressure, there are mathematical difficulties associated with some of these interpretations and currently it is considered that systolic pressure should be the primary focus of treatment in the elderly.

Genetics

The importance of genetic factors in the pathogenesis of essential hypertension is apparent in the similarity of blood pressure values between close relatives, such as siblings, and between parents and children. It has been suggested that there are several subtypes of hypertension, each with different pathogenetic mechanisms and different intermediate phenotypes, all of which result in the final phenotype of "essential hypertension". The problem has been that the phenotypic expression of different genotypes is complicated and often obscured by the interaction with other confounding factors. Thus, the application of therapeutic approaches founded upon phenotypic expression, such as plasma renin activity, has largely been unrewarding in the clinical practice setting. However, there can be no doubt that genetic components do play an important role in blood pressure regulation and this is well illustrated by the comparison of different racial groups.

Ethnicity

High blood pressure is a major health problem in African-American populations, with an estimated prevalence of about 25%. Considering that hypertension appears to be particularly difficult to control in African-American patients, this represents a considerable public health problem. Furthermore, the manifestations of uncontrolled hypertension are slightly different in African-American patients compared to their non-black counterparts. For example, the development of hypertensive renal failure is much more likely in African-Americans with hypertension compared to whites.[13]

In contrast, a different picture is seen in Westernized Asian communities, in whom hypertension is frequently associated with obesity, derangements of glucose and lipid metabolism, and type II diabetes mellitus – so-called "metabolic syndrome" or "insulin resistance".[14,15]

Aetiology of Hypertension

The aetiology of hypertension reflects a number of factors – genetic predisposition, environmental influences, iatrogenic causes and unknown components (Table 2).

Genetic factors

As discussed previously, genomics plays an important role in the development of hypertension and its CV consequences. The current view is that there are polygenic influences underlying the development of hypertension. In this respect, a number of "risk genotypes" probably exist, and these genotypes influence vascular tone, renal function, sodium homeostasis and activity of the renin–angiotensin system. Different permutations of these "risk genotypes" probably determine the severity of the hypertensive problem and, ultimately, the particular manifestation of atherosclerotic CV problems – coronary disease, cerebrovascular disease or peripheral vascular disease.

The aetiology of hypertension

Genetic predisposition
Environmental influences
- Obesity
- Salt
- Alcohol
- Smoking

Iatrogenic
- Corticosteroids
- Prednisolone
- Hormonal oral contraceptive
- Non-steroidal anti-inflammatory drugs

Unknown factors and unexplained interactions between known factors

Table 2. The aetiology of hypertension.

Sociological and dietary factors

Obesity

Obesity (and physical inactivity) are particularly important; obese people are more likely to develop hypertension than non-obese individuals. There is a well-established overlap between hypertension and other clinical features which have come to be known as the "metabolic syndrome" or "syndrome X" or "insulin resistance". Thus, hypertension, obesity (particularly central obesity), glucose intolerance and type II diabetes mellitus, dyslipidaemia (particularly with hypertriglyceridaemia and low high-density lipoprotein (HDL) cholesterol) have collectively been identified as part of the metabolic syndrome of insulin resistance.[15]

Salt

There is a variety of scientific information that relates an increase in salt intake with a rise in blood pressure. Population studies have found that the more salt a population consumes, the higher the average blood pressure. These studies and the resulting salt hypothesis receive further confirmation from observations that extreme salt loading can cause a rise in blood pressure.[16]

Alcohol

Most epidemiological studies have shown a significant positive correlation between alcohol consumption and blood pressure. There is also evidence for a correlation between a high alcohol intake and stroke mortality and morbidity. However, in contrast, lower blood pressures have been recorded in individuals who regularly consume modest amounts of alcohol (fewer than two alcoholic drinks per day) when compared to those who do not drink at all.[17]

Smoking

After acute smoking (one or two cigarettes) a pressor effect is observed, with blood pressure rising markedly. Despite this, epidemiological evidence shows no relationship between chronic cigarette smoking and blood pressure. However, smoking is a well-recognized and potent independent risk factor for coronary heart disease (CHD) and is closely associated with atheromatous renal artery stenosis.

Stress
As hypertension is more prevalent in developed societies, the hypothesis that stress may play a causative role in its development is plausible and attractive. In reality, most epidemiological studies seeking to evaluate a connection between stress and sustained hypertension have been negative or inconclusive.

Ambient temperature and seasonal variations in blood pressure
Blood pressure values are consistently higher in colder weather and hence in the winter months. In addition, there is less variation in blood pressure in areas where there is less seasonal variation in temperature.

Potassium
Epidemiological observations have indicated that a high average potassium intake is associated with a lower blood pressure. Therapeutic trials of potassium supplementation have individually given variable but usually negative results, although a meta-analysis did show a modest antihypertensive effect.[18]

Calcium
It has been suggested that calcium deficiency might play a role in the development of hypertension. However, several carefully conducted clinical trials have failed to show that calcium supplementation has any effect on blood pressure.[19]

Iatrogenic or "pharmacological"

The regular consumption of large quantities of alcohol is known to have a pressor effect (and it is also associated with an increased calorie intake), such that changing from a high alcohol intake to a lower intake has been shown to reduce blood pressure by about 5–10 mmHg.

With respect to specific drug treatments, non-steroidal anti-inflammatory drugs (NSAIDs), which the patient may acquire over the counter, are numerically the most important because they are particularly likely to interfere with the efficacy of antihypertensive drug treatment. Other drugs are known to predispose to the development of hypertension (e.g. corticosteroids, such as prednisone, and the oral contraceptive pill). Interestingly, however, the low-dose oestrogen preparations contained within oestrogen replacement therapy are not usually associated with any increase in blood pressure and, in fact, probably tend to reduce blood pressure.[20,21]

Even after taking account all the genetic and environmental influences discussed above, a large amount of variation of blood pressure between and within populations remains unexplained. Furthermore, although environmental influences may assume some significance on a population basis, it is often very difficult to quantify their direct relevance to the hypertension of an individual patient.

Prognosis in Hypertension

It is well established that high blood pressure is associated with premature CV morbidity and mortality. However, the ultimate outcome is determined not only by the blood pressure level itself, but also by the presence or absence of concomitant risk factors such as cigarette smoking, hypercholesterolaemia or type II diabetes mellitus (Figure 14).[22] The different combinations of different risk factors, allied to different genetic profiles and to different environmental influences, probably explain the differential death rates for coronary heart disease (CHD) and stroke seen in different individuals, different cultures and different countries.

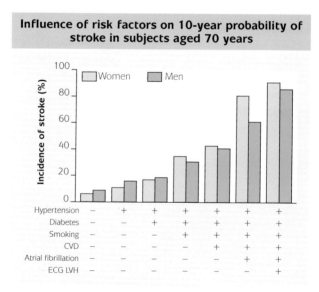

Figure 14. The influence of risk factors on the 10-year probability of stroke in subjects aged 70 years. Data from reference 22.

Untreated (uncontrolled) hypertension

The recognition of the importance of uncontrolled hypertension was first definitively documented in the data compiled by life assurance and actuarial companies.[23] This provided the evidence that higher blood pressures were associated with a reduction in life expectancy, at all ages and in both sexes. This was further reinforced by prospective observational studies, such as the Framingham study.[24] These studies defined the risk of higher blood pressures for CV morbidity and mortality with an increased frequency of stroke, coronary artery disease, cardiac failure, progressive renal disease and other vascular problems, such as dissecting aortic aneurysm.

In the middle half of the 20th century, there was considerable debate as to whether the CV risk conferred by high blood pressure

Hypertension and CHD mortality			
	6 year age-adjusted mortality males aged 35–57 years (MRFIT data)		
Systolic BP(mmHg)	n	Rate per 1000	Relative risk
<110	21,378	3.9	1.00
120	66,069	4.2	1.08
130	98,816	4.4	1.13
140	79,295	6.9	1.77
150	44,384	9.3	2.38
160	21,471	13.0	3.33
170	9,307	14.7	3.77
180	4,013	21.7	5.56
>180	3,190	24.9	6.38

Table 3. Event rates and blood pressure.

was graded or whether there was a threshold level of blood pressure at above which the risk became apparent. The seminal studies of McMahon, Collins, Peto and colleagues clearly summarize the problems of uncontrolled hypertension through their meta-analysis of nine major prospective observational studies involving 420,000 patients (see Figures 6 and 7). Their analysis conclusively demonstrated that the relationship between CVD and blood pressure (BP) is continuous, such that the risk of CV complications increases as the BP increases (probably from about 110/70 mmHg and above). In terms of absolute numbers, therefore, most CV and cerebrovascular events occur with BP values that many (in the past) would have considered to be "normal" (Table 3). This concept has been reinforced in a recent publication from Framingham in which high "normal" BP values are associated with poorer outcomes than low normal BP values in both men and women (Figures 15 and 16).[25]

As has been discussed previously, it is always important to appreciate the importance of the multiplicative adverse

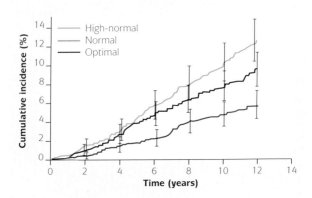

Figure 15. The impact of high normal blood pressure on the 10-year cumulative risk of cardiovascular disease in men. Data from reference 25.

effects of other risk factors, such as cigarette smoking or hyper-cholesterolaemia. The interactive increases associated with these factors (along with diabetes) in the 10-year risk of stroke and CHD in a 59-year-old man are shown in Figures 17 and 18, respectively.[26] The importance of other factors that may augment the CV risk at any given level of blood pressure should also be appreciated. For example, the presence of left ventricular hypertrophy, or the presence of established CV target organ damage (such as a previous stroke or myocardial infarction) confers a much greater adverse prognosis than that seen in the hypertensive patient with the same level of blood pressure in whom such target organ damage has not yet occurred.

Treated (controlled) hypertension

Much of the evidence demonstrating the benefit of antihypertensive therapy was derived from the early intervention trials of drug treatment, which were undertaken in the more severe

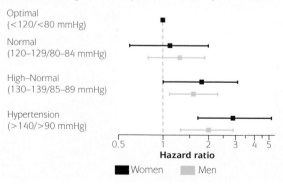

Figure 16. The relationship of blood pressure category to the risk of a major cardiovascular event in men and women. Data from reference 25.

Influence of risk factors on incidence of stroke

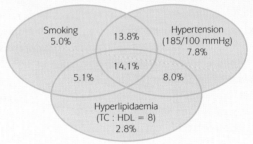

59-year-old man, non-smoker, BP 140/85 mmHg, TC : HDL = 4
10-year risk of stroke = 2.8%

Smoking
5.0%

13.8%

Hypertension
(185/100 mmHg)
7.8%

14.1%

5.1%

8.0%

Hyperlipidaemia
(TC : HDL = 8)
2.8%

All risk factors + diabetes = 21.7%

Figure 17. The influence of various risk factors on the incidence of stroke.

Influence of risk factors on incidence of CHD

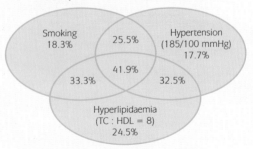

59-year-old man, non-smoker, BP 140/85 mmHg, TC : HDL = 4
10-year risk of CHD event = 11.9%

Smoking
18.3%

25.5%

Hypertension
(185/100 mmHg)
17.7%

41.9%

33.3%

32.5%

Hyperlipidaemia
(TC : HDL = 8)
24.5%

All risk factors + diabetes = 47.9%

Figure 18. The effect of various risk factors on the incidence of CHD.

forms of hypertension, including malignant (or accelerated) phase hypertension. These trials produced unequivocal evidence that antihypertensive treatment was beneficial.

Severe hypertension
In untreated individuals, mortality from severe or malignant phase hypertension approached 100% in 2 years. With the advent of antihypertensive drug treatment, this fell to about 50% and, in modern therapeutic practice, patients with malignant hypertension should now have a 2-year mortality of less than 5%.[27]

Moderate hypertension
In the 1960s, the outcome studies were extended to those patients with moderately severe hypertension, and these showed that most of the CV consequences, particularly stroke, cardiac failure and renal failure, could be significantly reduced. The impact on coronary artery disease (myocardial infarction and sudden cardiac death), however, was relatively disappointing.[28]

Mild hypertension
The outcome benefits of treating mild hypertension have been explored more recently, leading to the conclusion that the reduction of blood pressure in patients with diastolic blood pressure in the range 90–105 mmHg conferred benefit, particularly by reducing the incidence of stroke. The impact on events related to coronary artery disease, although beneficial, remains less than predicted (Figure 19).[29]

Randomized placebo-controlled outcome trials
In the 1980s and the early years of the 1990s, a series of placebo-controlled trials were performed in a large number of patients with mild to moderate (Stage I to II) hypertension. Although in specific details these trials differed in the populations that were studied and the benefits that were achieved, all were able to show, to a greater or lesser extent, statistically significant reductions in CV events. The definitive evidence from these

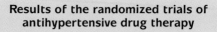

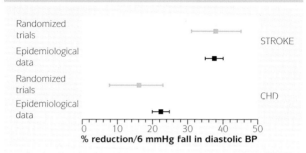

Figure 19. Summarizing results of the randomized trials of antihypertensive drug therapy: comparison of the randomized trial and the reductions anticipated from epidemiological data. Data from reference 29.

trials was summarized in the meta-analysis of McMahon, Collins, Peto and colleagues (Figure 20).

 Their analysis was conclusively able to show that, in a population, a modest reduction in diastolic blood pressure (by about 6 mmHg on average) was associated with a 38% reduction in stroke events and a 16% reduction in CHD events. The reduction in stroke events was closely similar to that predicted from the epidemiological studies (up to 40%), whereas in coronary artery disease there was a shortfall relative to the predicted 20–25% reduction. There is no definitive explanation for this "shortfall" in CHD prevention, but the likeliest explanation appears to lie in the duration of antihypertensive drug treatment and the relatively short-term nature of the trials contributing to the meta-analysis. It is also interesting to note that in these trials the incidence of CHD exceeded that of stroke (Figure 20), a pattern which has not been apparent in recent trials where the incidence of stroke predominates. Furthermore, coronary disease development is closely associated with dyslipidaemia,

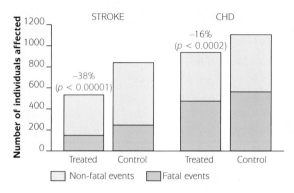

Figure 20. Randomized control trials in hypertension: reductions in cardiovascular events. Data from reference 29.

diabetic control and smoking, three risk factors that were not addressed or managed aggressively in the earlier hypertension trials.

Recent trials which are reviewed later in this book have served to reinforce the fact that the prognosis of the hypertensive patient is determined not only by the level of blood pressure itself, but also by the age and sex of the patient; the presence or absence of coexisting risk factors for CVD (particularly disorders of glucose or lipid metabolism); and whether or not the patient has pre-existing target organ damage. Nevertheless, the adverse prognosis associated with hypertension can be positively influenced by antihypertensive drug treatment, such that the better the BP control, the better the eventual outcome, with significantly reduced CV morbidity and mortality.

Management of Patients with Hypertension

Clinical features

Most patients with hypertension do not have any symptoms directly attributable to the raised blood pressure itself but, occasionally, in no more than about 5% of patients, the initial clinical history and examination may reveal clues to a possible underlying cause (Table 4). For example, a phaeochromo-cytoma might be suspected if there is a history of episodes of palpitations and sweating associated with high blood pressure values (when normal blood pressure values are obtained at other, asymptomatic times): alternatively, a systolic–diastolic bruit on abdominal examination might indicate underlying renal artery stenosis.

The clinical history, therefore, rarely provides information which is of direct relevance to the cause of the hypertension itself. Instead, the clinical history usually seeks to identify other

Causes of elevated blood pressure
Primary hypertension (90–95%) Also termed "idiopathic" or "essential" hypertension

Secondary hypertension (about 5% of cases)
Renal or renovascular disease
Endocrine disease
  • Phaeochromocytoma (catecholamine excess)
  • Hyperaldosteronism (including Conn's syndrome)
  • Cushing's syndrome (corticosteroid excess)
  • Acromegaly and hypothyroidism
Coarctation of the aorta
Iatrogenic
  • Hormonal oral contraceptive
  • Non-steroidal anti-inflammatory drugs

Table 4. Causes of elevated blood pressure.

factors which might contribute to the overall CV risk of the patient: for example, cigarette and alcohol consumption; family history of hypertension, or diabetes, or premature CVD in a first-degree relative. There may also be a history of arthritis and the use of NSAIDs or hypertension in association with the hormonal oral contraceptive.

Correspondingly, in the absence of specific clues, only a limited amount of useful information can be gleaned from the routine clinical examination. Often overlooked, however, is fundoscopy: a quick and simple assessment of the duration and/or severity of the hypertension via the appearance of the retinal vasculature.

Clinical investigations

Routine investigation for all patients with hypertension
In addition to a standard clinical history and examination, the following routine laboratory evaluations constitute the recommended basic "work-up" in both the primary and secondary healthcare settings.

- Urinalysis. The identification of proteinuria and microscopic haematuria by a simple "dipstix" test of urine may indicate some degree of renal arteriolar necrosis and nephrosclerosis, even in patients with non-malignant hypertension. Alternatively, they may indicate underlying intrinsic renal disease, such as diabetic nephropathy, polycystic kidney disease, chronic pyelonephritis or chronic glomerulonephritis (particularly IgA nephropathy).

- Serum chemistry. Abnormal sodium and potassium levels are particularly important. For example, high sodium and low potassium may indicate primary hyperaldosteronism. In patients already receiving drug treatment, however, it is important to remember that drug-induced electrolyte changes occur with angiotensin-converting enzyme inhibitors (ACEIs) or angiotensin II antagonists (particularly in combination with potassium-sparing agents), and also with all types of diuretics.

- Blood urea nitrogen and serum creatinine concentrations. These are simple indices of renal function. High levels suggest either that the hypertension has caused a degree of renal impairment or that an underlying renal disease may be creating or worsening the hypertension.

- Lipid profiles and glucose concentrations. These are integral to the calculation of the absolute CV risk status for each individual patient.
- Cardiac status. A standard 12-lead ECG constitutes a baseline against which any later ECG changes can be compared. It may also provide information about underlying ischaemic heart disease and/or the presence of left ventricular (LV) hypertrophy.

The chest X-ray is no longer considered useful for assessing cardiac size in terms of LV hypertrophy. In fact, neither the ECG nor the chest radiograph are particularly sensitive measures of LV size. Nevertheless, the detection of LV hypertrophy with strain pattern on the ECG is a particularly adverse prognostic indicator (Figure 21).

In a patient with borderline clinical blood pressure readings, the presence or absence of LV hypertrophy can also be a useful guide to the need for antihypertensive treatment. For this reason, echocardiography is currently the preferred method for assessing LV size (and function) and is increasingly becoming part of the routine work-up in specialist hypertension clinics.

LVH and strain

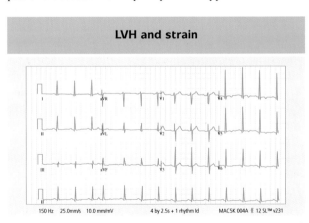

Figure 21. An ECG showing left ventricular hypertrophy and "strain" pattern. Reproduced with permission from Lip GYH, Chung N. *Hypertension: patients at risk*. London: Elsevier, 2002.

Additional investigations

The following investigations are not part of the routine work-up but may be indicated in response to clinical clues or via abnormal results from the basic investigations (Table 5).

24-hour urine chemistries

Different analyses can clarify particular issues: e.g. aldosterone in suspected primary aldosteronism, catecholamine and its metabolites (e.g. metanephrines, vanillyl mandelic acid) in suspected phaeochromocytoma; urinary free cortisol (allied to plasma cortisol profiles) in Cushing's syndrome; quantification of creatinine clearance and protein output in renal impairment or diabetic nephropathy.

Imaging techniques

Ultrasonography of the kidneys is the preferred screening test capable of identifying hydronephrosis, polycystic kidneys or diminished renal size.

For renal artery stenosis, however, routine ultrasonography is not sufficiently sensitive and, though the detection rate is improved by Doppler ultrasound examination, the definitive test when there is a high index of suspicion is still renal arteriography. There is not yet an agreed, definitive non-invasive screening test: some authorities continue to recommend renography with and without an ACEI, but magnetic resonance angiography is proving increasingly useful and is probably the most sensitive non-invasive test.

Indications for further investigations

Malignant/accelerated phase hypertension
Resistant hypertension
Young patient (especially <25 years – optionally <40 years)
"Unusual" clinical history/examination
Abnormality detected by routine screening tests

Table 5. Indications for further investigations.

Radionuclide imaging using 131I-labelled meta-iodo-benzylguanadine may be useful for localizing phaeochromocytoma, but it is a costly and time-consuming test and requires a substantial amount of expertise to interpret. Abdominal ultrasound or CT scanning may occasionally show adrenal tumours but, increasingly, MRI is proving diagnostically superior in detecting adrenal tumours that may be associated with hyperaldosteronism or phaeochromocytoma.

Hormone measurement

Plasma levels, often in conjunction with urinary measurements, may be useful in confirming the diagnosis of an endocrine cause:

- Primary hyperaldosteronism (Conn's syndrome) – increased plasma aldosterone and suppressed plasma renin activity.
- Secondary hyperaldosteronism – increased plasma aldosterone and increased plasma renin activity; it is important that these measurements are obtained from a fasting patient who is supine (preferable before rising in the morning).
- Phaeochromocytoma – increased plasma norepinephrine, epinephrine and dopamine, and increased 24-hour urinary catecholamine metabolite output.
- Cushing's syndrome – plasma cortisol and adrenocorticotrophin concentration profiles and urinary free cortisol measurements may be helpful.
- Acromegaly and hypothyroidism – plasma concentrations of intact growth hormone and thyroxin (or thyroid-stimulating hormone), respectively.

Cardiovascular risk assessment

Most of the current major guidelines for the treatment of hypertension acknowledge the importance of the interaction of high blood pressure with other risk factors. The current Joint National Committee (JNC) guidelines,[30] in concert with current strategies for the prevention of CVD in general and CHD in particular, have focused on overall risk as a determinant of the treatment intervention priorities. Thus, the "risk" associated with a confirmed clinical blood pressure of 150/96 mmHg will vary according to the patient's age, gender, smoking habit, presence/absence of diabetes mellitus and so forth. A number of charts, algorithms, computer programs, etc. are available for calculating the 10-year risk of CHD. The Coronary Risk Prediction Charts produced by the Joint British Societies (British Cardiac Society, British Hypertension Society, British Hyperlipidaemia Association and British Diabetic Association) are shown in Figure 22. Since risk is variable and since the absolute benefit of treatment is variable, blood pressure values are no longer considered entirely in isolation. The situation is further complicated by issues related to drug costs, cost-effectiveness, patient numbers, etc. The current guidelines from the British Hypertension Society (BHS) illustrate this concept. In brief summary, the current BHS guidelines recommend that a confirmed BP of 160/100 mmHg or above warrants antihypertensive drug treatment, whereas 140/90 mmHg and above, although hypertension by definition, warrants antihypertensive drug treatment only when the 10-year CHD risk exceeds 15% (or when there is evidence of prior CVD or target organ damage) (Table 6).[30] There is some confusion between CHD risk and CVD risk but, not surprisingly, there is a high correlation between CHD risk and CVD risk, and a 10-year CHD risk threshold of ≥15% is equivalent to a 10-year

BHS treatment guidelines

Blood Pressure: 140–159 mmHg and/or 90–99 mmHg Recommendations

1. Target organ damage
   Rx: drug treatment
2. Other CV risk factors and 10-year CHD risk >15%
   Rx: (a) Lifestyle measures (up to 6/12)
       (b) Drug treatment
3. No other risk factors and 10-year CHD risk <15%
   Rx: (a) Lifestyle measures (up to 12/12)
       (b) Reassess annually

Table 6. BHS guidelines and CHD risk.

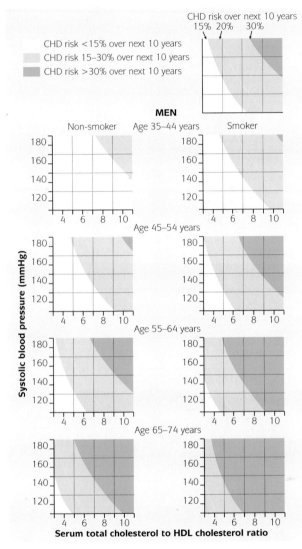

Figure 22a. Coronary risk prediction charts for men and women without diabetes. Reproduced with permission from Ramsay LE, Williams B, Johnston GD *et al.* Guidelines for management of hypertension: report of the third working party of the British Hypertension Society. *J Hum Hypertens* 1999; **13**: 569–592.

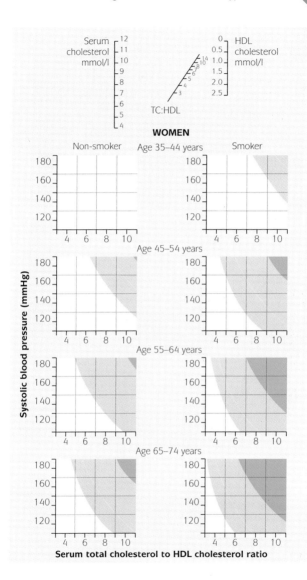

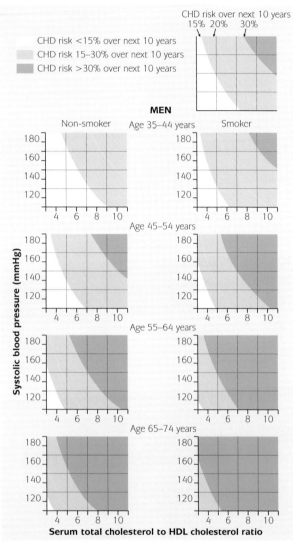

Figure 22b. Coronary risk prediction charts for men and women with diabetes. Reproduced with permission from Ramsay LE, Williams B, Johnston GD *et al.* Guidelines for management of hypertension: report of the third working party of the British Hypertension Society. *J Hum Hypertens* 1999; **13**: 569–592.

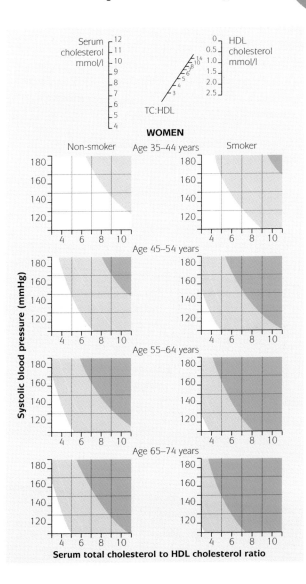

Serum cholesterol mmol/l
12
11
10
9
8
7
6
5
4

HDL cholesterol mmol/l
0
0.5
1.0
1.5
2.0
2.5

TC:HDL
14
10
8
6
5
4
3

WOMEN

Age 35–44 years
Non-smoker   Smoker

Age 45–54 years

Age 55–64 years

Age 65–74 years

Systolic blood pressure (mmHg)

Serum total cholesterol to HDL cholesterol ratio

CVD risk of ≥20%, on average. Calculation of CHD risk and CVD risk separately for each patient is laborious and the evidence suggests that targeting CHD risk for antihypertensive therapy is preferable, and simpler, accepting that this entails some minor inaccuracy in the risk calculation and the targeting of treatment.

24-hour ambulatory blood pressure measurement

Our current understanding of the long-term adverse CV consequences of uncontrolled hypertension and the benefits of antihypertensive drug treatment is derived from conventional clinical BP measurements. However, the limitations of conventional blood pressure measurement and the prognostic superiority of 24-hour blood pressure measurements (Figure 23) have been recognized increasingly since Sokolow *et al.* first demonstrated in 1966 that ambulatory blood pressure measurements were highly predictive of CV risk (in terms of heart attack, stroke and death).[31] More recent studies have

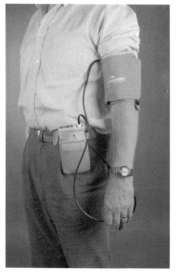

Figure 23. A 24-hour blood pressure monitor.

demonstrated consistently that the values derived from 24-hour measurements are more closely correlated with CV target organ damage than conventional clinical blood pressure (Figure 24 and Table 7).[32]

Which patients should be monitored?

Although it remains the subject of debate, constraints on time, resources and finances mean that there is not yet a place for

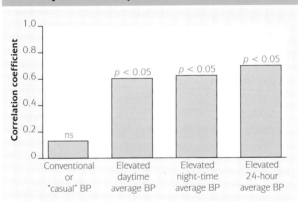

Correlations between LV mass index and elevated systolic blood pressure measurement

Figure 24. The correlation of elevated blood pressure and left ventricular mass. Reproduced with permission from White *et al.* (1994).

24-hour blood pressure correlates with different types of target organ damage

Overall target organ damage score
Left ventricular mass
Impaired left ventricular function
(Micro)albuminuria
Brain damage (cerebral lacunae)
Retinopathy
Intima media thickness (carotid)

Table 7. 24-hour blood pressure correlates with different types of target organ damage.

24-hour blood pressure measurement in the routine work-up of every hypertensive patient. Thus, outside of the research environment, the current consensus is that 24-hour blood pressure monitoring should be reserved for specialists and/or specific clinical circumstances, particularly where there are potential management issues.[8,32]

- "White coat" hypertension (i.e. a rise in blood pressure associated with the procedure of blood pressure measurement) is common, and in some patients this increase is sufficient to consistently elevate the measured blood pressure into the hypertensive range. The mechanism underlying "white coat" (alternative terminology: "isolated clinical hypertension") hypertension is unknown, but up to 20% of patients diagnosed as hypertensive according to clinical blood pressure measurements may not actually fulfil the criteria for hypertension according to their 24-hour blood pressure measurement, with average daytime values of less than 130/80 mmHg. At present, there is no evidence to warrant early drug treatment in patients who clearly have "white coat" hypertension. There remains considerable debate, however, about the patient with hypertension according to clinical measurements, but an average daytime ambulatory blood pressure in the ranges 130–140 mmHg systolic and 80–90 mmHg diastolic is usually considered as hypertensive.

- Borderline hypertension. 24-hour blood pressure measurement may help to clarify the diagnosis and the need for treatment, especially in those where target organ involvement is suggested on physical examination.

- Resistant hypertension. Assuming that there are no problems with compliance, patients with resistant hypertension are those who fail to respond satisfactorily to multiple drugs and combination regimens. Before embarking on further investigation in search of underlying cause, 24-hour blood pressure monitoring may identify patients who have a "white coat" response when their blood pressure is checked at follow-up.

Limitations of 24-hour ambulatory blood pressure monitoring

The usefulness of the values derived from 24-hour ambulatory blood pressure monitoring (ABPM) is compromised by the absence of a universally agreed normal range for blood pressure (as measured by this technique). According to conventional clinical BP criteria, and according to which set of guidelines is adopted, the upper limit of normal clinical blood pressure is generally accepted as 140/90 mmHg. Data from recent studies are consistent, however, in showing that this level is "high" if applied to the calculated average 24-hour values, which typically show that normal daytime ambulatory values fall in the range of 120–130 mmHg for systolic blood pressure and 70–80 mmHg for diastolic blood pressure. Correspondingly, the BP targets for treatment are lower for ABPM values than for conventional clinic values (Table 8).

There are no outcome studies in which the management of the patient has been guided according to 24-hour blood pressure values. At present, therefore, clinical blood pressure values remain the "gold standard" for most management decisions in routine clinical practice.

General management – the principles

Should isolated systolic hypertension be treated?

Isolated systolic hypertension (ISH) is defined as an elevated systolic blood pressure above 160 mmHg with an associated

Blood pressure treatment targets				
	Clinic BP (mmHg)		Mean daytime ABPM (mmHg)	
	No Diabetes	Diabetes	No Diabetes	Diabetes
Optimal BP	<140/85	<140/80	<130/80	<130/75
Audit standard	<150/90	<140/85	<140/85	<140/80

Table 8. Blood pressure treatment targets.

normal diastolic blood pressure of less than 90 mmHg. It is now clear, however, that in any age group, systolic blood pressure is a more consistent predictor of CV risk than diastolic blood pressure and treatment is therefore warranted.

The SHEP study (Systolic Hypertension in the Elderly Programme) was the first to address specifically the issue of whether treatment was indicated for ISH; previously there were concerns that reduction of an isolated systolic pressure might actually be harmful.[33] The results of SHEP (and other studies) have shown clear benefits with reduction in CV morbidity and mortality, and this is illustrated by the meta-analysis of these trials (Figure 25).[34]

The current recommendations from the JNC and BHS endorse these findings – elderly patients should be treated if they are found to have a confirmed systolic blood pressure above 160 mmHg, regardless of the diastolic blood pressure level.

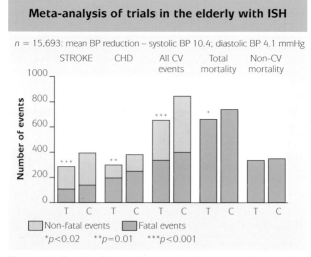

Figure 25. Results of the meta-analysis of trials in the elderly with isolated systolic hypertension. Reproduced with permission from Elsevier Science from Staessen JA, Gasowski J, Wang JG et al. Risks of untreated systolic hypertension in the elderly: meta-analysis of outcome trials. *Lancet* 2000; **355**: 865–872.[34]

How far should blood pressure be lowered?

In some studies, particularly post-hoc analyses involving relatively small patient numbers, a relationship has been identified between low diastolic blood pressure and increased CV risk. These findings have led to the concept of a "J-curve" (albeit with a wide range of different cut-off values for diastolic blood pressure in the different studies), whereby excessive blood pressure reduction might actually be harmful, particularly if there is underlying coronary artery disease. The putative mechanism is that excessive blood pressure reduction compromises diastolic filling of the coronary arteries and therefore predisposes patients to myocardial ischaemia and/or infarction. However, these mechanistic concerns have not been confirmed in any prospective evaluation.

The SHEP study provided evidence against the J-curve concept. Elderly patients with pre-existing coronary disease are obviously at high CV risk; in the SHEP study, patients had average diastolic blood pressure reduced to 70 mmHg, leading to a 25% reduction in the number of coronary events, despite 61% of these patients having abnormal ECGs at baseline and 5% having a history of myocardial infarction (MI). More recently, the results of the Hypertension Optimal Treatment (HOT) study were similarly reassuring, with no increase in adverse outcomes in patients targeted to diastolic BP control of less than 80 mmHg, compared to those targeted to less than 90 mmHg.[35] These results do not constitute definitive proof, but they reinforce the concept that there is no lower diastolic blood pressure level at which risk is increased by blood pressure reduction, provided that the blood pressure reduction is achieved gradually and progressively in high-risk patients.

Management of uncomplicated hypertensive patients

In the asymptomatic patient with no significant concomitant disease, a range of drugs is available for the patient whose hypertension has not responded to lifestyle measures (i.e. weight reduction, reduced alcohol consumption, regular physical exercise and sodium intake restriction). There is now a clear departure from the rigid stepped-care approach based on thiazide diuretics and beta-blockers. The concept of individualized treatment is "fashionable" but it is essentially an extension of conventional clinical practice, whereby negative factors often influence the drug choice. Thus, beta-blockers are avoided in a patient known to have obstructive airways disease, a thiazide diuretic is not usually prescribed for a patient with a history of gout, and an ACEI is not the treatment of choice in a patient with widespread peripheral vascular disease and possible renovascular problems.

Management of patients with concomitant disease

Concomitant disease and/or concurrent drug treatments are potentially complicating factors in a significant number of hypertensive patients.

Diabetes mellitus

Hypertension occurs in about 20% of patients with insulin-dependent diabetes mellitus and 30–50% of patients with non-insulin-dependent diabetes mellitus; optimal blood pressure control is a priority in these patients.

Traditionally, it was recommended that thiazide diuretics were best avoided in view of their potentially adverse metabolic effects (e.g. insulin resistance) and that beta-blockers may occasionally cause problems in the "brittle" diabetic patient by masking the premonitory symptoms of insulin-induced hypoglycaemia. These are not compelling contraindications in routine clinical practice, but there is currently a clear preference for the use of ACEI drugs (and/or angiotensin receptor blockers).

ACEIs or angiotensin II receptor blockers are now generally regarded as first-line treatment for patients with hypertension and diabetes, with or without microalbuminuria or in those patients with more advanced renal disease. There is good evidence from clinical trials of the effectiveness of these agents in reducing microalbuminuria and there is also substantial evidence that blockade of the renin–angiotensin system with angiotensin II receptor blockers retards the decline in renal function by mechanisms other than blood pressure reduction.

At present, however, to make an impact on macrovascular events such as MI and stroke, the emphasis in the treatment of the hypertensive diabetic is on achieving optimal blood pressure control (i.e. a target of less than 130/80 mmHg), usually by means of blockade of the renin–angiotensin system as the basis of the treatment regimen. To achieve this level of BP, multiple antihypertensive drug treatments will be required: this will usually require that calcium channel blockers (CCBs) and other drugs, including diuretics, be added.

Dyslipidaemia

The minor dyslipidaemic effects of thiazide diuretics (increases in both cholesterol and triglycerides) and beta-blockers (increases in triglycerides and decreases in HDL cholesterol) are widely recognized but are of debatable clinical significance. The calcium antagonists and ACEIs are lipid neutral and the alpha-blocker group remains the only antihypertensive drug class for which there is evidence of a beneficial effect on lipid profile.

Selective alpha-1-blockers (e.g. doxazosin) have been associated with small reductions (about 5–10%) in total cholesterol. For this reason (though the magnitude of the effect is relatively small), some physicians consider alpha-blockers to be the drug of choice for hypertensive patients with background metabolic abnormalities such as mild hypercholesterolaemia (or glucose intolerance). However, the results of the ALLHAT study would dispute this, since in this trial doxazosin as a first-line therapy was associated with a two-fold increase in the incidence of congestive heart failure and a 20% increase in the risk of stroke compared to the diuretic treatment arm.

Symptomatic coronary artery disease

In the absence of contraindications, beta-blockers, which have both antihypertensive and anti-ischaemic activity, are the first-line treatment in the patient with hypertension and angina. If a second drug is required, either for reducing blood pressure or for the prevention of extertional angina, a long-acting, once-daily dihydropyridine calcium antagonist should be added.

If beta-blockers are contraindicated or poorly tolerated, long-acting formulations of the non-dihydropyridine calcium antagonists verapamil or diltiazem are the preferred types of anti-anginal and antihypertensive monotherapy.

Post-stroke

Despite the wealth of data confirming the benefits of antihypertensive drug treatment as a primary prevention strategy for stroke, it is only recently that the benefits of a secondary prevention strategy have been confirmed by prospective outcome trials.

In the HOPE study (with ramipril)[36] and in the PROGRESS study (with perindopril–indapamide),[37] there were significant reductions in stroke events in patients known to be at high CV risk. Of particular interest was the PROGRESS study, in which post-stroke patients, whether normotensive or hypertensive, benefited from treatment (Figure 26). Although the subject of some debate, the benefits in this high-risk patient group appear

PROGRESS
Combination versus single drug therapy

Combination therapy (12/5 mmHg) and single drug therapy (5/3 mmHg)

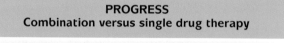

	Events active placebo			Risk reduction (95% CI)
Stroke		Favours active	Favours placebo	
Combination	150 255			43% (30 to54%)
Single drug	157 165			5% (–19 to 23%)
Total	307 420			28% (17 to38%)
Major vascular events				
Combination	231 367			40% (29 to 49%)
Single drug	227 237			4% (–15 to 20%)
Total	458 604			26% (16 to 34%)

0.5   1.0   1.5
Hazard ratio
Tests for homogeneity (combination versus single drug): both <0.001

Figure 26. Results of the PROGRESS trial demonstrating the benefits associated with treatment in patients who had previously suffered a stroke. Reproduced with permission of Elsevier Science from reference 37.

to be directly related to BP reduction rather than the pharmacological characteristics of any particular drug type.

Arthritic conditions

The concurrent use of NSAIDs, including some of the new cyclo-oxygenase-2 (COX-2)-specific inhibitors, rather than arthritis itself, can interfere with the effectiveness of several different types of antihypertensive agent. In particular, the efficacy of loop diuretics, beta-blockers and ACEIs is most likely to be compromised, and that of calcium antagonists and alpha-1 antagonists is least likely to be affected.

Management of "special" populations of hypertensives
The elderly

The number of people over the age of 65 years continues to increase. In most societies, blood pressure increases with age and elevated levels of blood pressure are common in the elderly. Elderly patients with hypertension are often difficult to manage. Pathophysiological changes associated with ageing are also associated with long-standing, uncontrolled hypertension. Diagnosis may not be straightforward and the incidence of concomitant disease will be higher than in younger patients. The preventative benefits of antihypertensive therapy in the elderly is well established (Figure 25) and treatment of hypertension is of greatest value in older patients who, because of additional risk factors or prevalent CVD, are at a higher risk of suffering a CV event. Several intervention trials have confirmed lower CVD risk in hypertensive patients aged into their early eighties when treated with a variety of antihypertensive drugs. Whilst there is some limited evidence to suggest that beta-blockers may not be as effective as thiazide diuretics in reducing CHD or total mortality in the elderly, thiazides alone or in combination with beta-blockers appear to be as effective as newer agents such as ACEIs and calcium antagonists. However, it should be appreciated that the benefits of treatment in the elderly are based upon the evidence from randomized controlled trials in selected patient groups, which may not be universally applicable to many elderly hypertensives. Thus, the treatment of hypertension in the elderly should be based upon an individualized approach, which inevitably cannot be strictly evidence based. There was no evidence from any of these trials that blood pressure reduction in the elderly was associated with any deleterious effects, with no excess of postural hypotension or symptomatic dizziness. Whilst the benefits of treating the elderly hypertensive are well established, some issues remain questionable in relation to treating the very elderly. No large outcome study has so far reported exclusively on hypertension in patients aged over 80 years, even though a number of studies have included such patients. A meta-analysis of these studies has demonstrated a significant benefit in reduction of stroke, CV events and heart failure, although total mortality was not reduced (Figure 27).[38] Furthermore, the potential benefits beyond blood pressure control that may be afforded by newer antihypertensive agents also require formal evaluation.

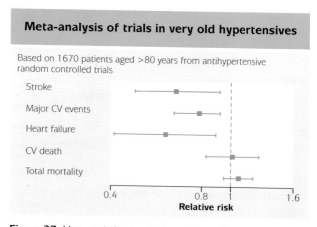

Meta-analysis of trials in very old hypertensives

Based on 1670 patients aged >80 years from antihypertensive random controlled trials

Figure 27. Meta-analysis of patients aged over 80 years who were enrolled in randomized outcome trials. Reproduced with permission from Elsevier Science from Gueyffier F, Bulpitt C, Boisel JP *et al.* for the INDANA Group. Antihypertensive drugs in very old people: a subgroup meta-analysis of randomised controlled trials. *Lancet* 1999; **353**: 793–796.[38]

Children and adolescents

Although only a tiny minority of children require antihypertensive drug therapy, long-term follow-up studies of cohorts of normal infants in children strongly suggest that the origins of adult essential hypertension are to be found in early childhood or even in the antenatal period. Children who are diagnosed as hypertensive usually have identifiable renovascular abnormalities requiring detailed and specialist management. The drug treatment of childhood hypertension has been hampered by several factors, including a lack of rigorous data about pharmacokinetics in children, age-related differences in drug response and the absence of appropriate drug formulations, and a lack of manufacturers' recommendations for the use of antihypertensive drugs in children. The latter problem may well be appropriately addressed in the future as the FDA in the USA has been mandated to identify drugs with potential health benefits in children and request that manufacturers conduct paediatric trials, with the incentive of an extension of overall patent life. The promulgation of this legislation is sufficiently recent that it has not yet had a major impact in promoting paediatric trials of antihypertensive agents. Thus, reliance must be placed on less well-controlled studies which, overall, indicate that the treatment of children and adolescents should be based upon the same rules as apply to the adult hypertensive population. Thus, all first-line antihypertensive agents appear to be appropriate and the doses should be given in a weight-related manner, in line with those recommended for adults.

Pregnancy-related hypertension

Hypertension in pregnancy should not be considered as a single entity and can be classified in a number of different ways:

- Chronic hypertension, which complicates between 1% and 5% of pregnancies, is normally defined as a blood pressure greater than 140/90 mmHg, and either predates the pregnancy or develops before 20 weeks gestation.
- Pregnancy-induced hypertension, which develops after 20 weeks of gestation and complicates 5–10% of pregnancies.

• Pre-eclampsia, which is pregnancy-induced hypertension associated with proteinuria or oedema or both, and virtually any organ system may be affected.

The types of hypertension in pregnancy differ primarily in the incidence, and not the nature, of maternal and perinatal complications; hypertension in pregnancy is consistently associated with an excess maternal mortality due to intracerebral haemorrhage, eclampsia or end organ dysfunction. Perinatal mortality and morbidity reflect both the foetal syndrome of pre-eclampsia (intra-uterine growth restriction) and the consequences of iatrogenic prematurity resulting from deteriorating maternal disease of foetal condition.

The management of hypertensive disease during pregnancy is a challenging problem for the physician, largely due to the relative paucity of therapeutic trial data on which to make clinical decisions. "Conventional" non-pharmacological strategies may not be applicable for hypertension during pregnancy. Thus, weight reduction and exercise would not normally be encouraged during pregnancy, and indeed bed rest is a means of improving utero-placental blood flow during pregnancy and is routine therapy in pre-eclampsia by maternal–foetal medicine specialists. However, appropriate dietary advice and strong discouragement of alcohol and tobacco use during pregnancy are of paramount importance.

The goal of treatment of hypertension in pregnancy is the reduction of both maternal and foetal risk. Thus, selection of therapy should be based not only on the antihypertensive efficacy of any drug, but also on the acute and long-term effects of these drugs on foetal well-being. Based on these criteria, alpha-methyldopa would be a common first choice of agent for treating hypertension in pregnancy. However, methyldopa may prove to be ineffective or poorly tolerated, in which instance alternative therapy must be considered. The use of diuretics in pregnancy is somewhat controversial based on the concern that pre-eclampsia is associated with a reduction of plasma volume and that foetal outcome is worse in chronically hypertensive women who fail to expand plasma volume. Despite these theoretical concerns, the evidence suggests that diuretics are not contraindicated in pregnancy, except where utero-placental perfusion is already reduced (diuretics are rarely, if ever, used in pregnancy hypertension in the USA).

There is evidence that the combined alpha- and beta-adrenoceptor blocking agent labetalol is relatively safe and effective in pregnancy. Other studies have suggested equal effectiveness for "pure" beta-blockers, but there is concern that whilst treatment may benefit the mother, the impact on maternal outcomes is less clear, particularly for atenolol.

The evidence regarding the safety and efficacy of CCBs in the treatment of hypertension in pregnancy is somewhat limited, thus their use in pregnancy has tended to be limited to either add-on therapy or where other drugs were contraindicated or not tolerated.

Finally, the use of ACEIs and angiotensin receptor blockers is considered to be absolutely contraindicated. These are known to reduce uterine blood flow and foetal survival in experimental animals, and thus they should also be avoided in patients who are planning to become pregnant.

Summary and conclusions

1. Investigation. Beyond the basic clinical "work-up", further screening investigations (in the absence of "clues" or pointers) are seldom fruitful and definitely not cost-effective.

2. 24-hour ABPM. In routine clinical practice – as distinct from clinical research – this technique is of limited applicability. It should only be used when the result will significantly alter the management of the patient. For example, the deliberate decision not to prescribe a drug treatment for a patient with a confirmed clinical BP of 158/98 mmHg because the 10-year CHD risk is less than 15% and, perhaps more importantly, because the daytime ABPM average is completely normal at less than 130/80 mmHg.

3. Treatment. There is clear evidence that antihypertensive drug treatment is beneficial in reducing CV morbidity and mortality. At present, the recommended treatment targets are less than 140/85 mmHg for uncomplicated hypertensive patients and less than 130/80 mmHg in diabetic patients.

Treatment of Hypertension

General principles

Although this section focuses upon the specific aspects of antihypertensive drug treatment, it is important to bear in mind that the level of blood pressure and its reduction is essentially a "surrogate end-point". The primary aim is reduction of overall CVD and CHD risk, for which blood pressure reduction is an evidence-based strategy. The current recommendations are that patients with a 10-year CHD risk of 15% or more are "eligible" for antihypertensive drug treatment as a primary prevention strategy, even with a relatively mild hypertension in the range 140–150 for systolic and 90–99 mmHg for diastolic BP. Overall, the treatment strategy should initially involve lifestyle intervention (or non-pharmacological treatment) with the addition of antihypertensive drug treatment where blood pressure control remains sub-optimal. The various guidelines suggest that the choice of the specific drug treatment should be based upon the compelling indications and contraindications of a particular drug class, which take account of specific patient characteristics, including other risk factors and co-morbidities. In reality, it is the compelling contraindications that tend to assume greater importance in drug selection.

Lifestyle modification

In a few patients, effective and sustained lifestyle modification will be sufficient to reduce blood pressure and/or CV risk to acceptable values. The recommended lifestyle measures are discussed in detail elsewhere, but the principal factors can be briefly summarized as follows:

- Cessation of smoking.
- Weight reduction to achieve an ideal body weight – in particular, via a reduced fat and total calorie intake.
- Regular dynamic physical exercise, such as brisk walking or regular swimming.

- Alcohol consumption limited for men to not more than 21 units and for women to not more than 14 units per week (this probably should be based on Body Mass Index, not on gender).
- Reduction in salt consumption.

A number of trials have sought to demonstrate the benefits of lifestyle modification in reducing blood pressure. In particular, attention has focused on the benefits of dietary salt reduction. Most of these studies have suggested that a moderate reduction in sodium consumption reduces blood pressure to a small extent. Furthermore, in the recent Dietary Approaches to Stop Hypertension (DASH) study, which assessed the benefits of a diet rich in fresh fruits, vegetables and low-fat dairy products, the lower the salt intake, the lower was the blood pressure.[39] Achieving lifestyle modification is never easy, but in the setting of a controlled trial it certainly can be attained. The Trial Of Non-pharmacological interventions in the Elderly (TONE) documented that lifestyle modifications, weight reduction and reduced sodium intake could be achieved in elderly patients.[40]

It is often argued that the benefits associated with lifestyle modifications are relatively modest and relatively expensive, in that they can often only be achieved when considerable support is provided by way of frequent clinic visits. Nonetheless, small blood pressure reductions in populations as a whole can have a substantial impact in reducing strokes, heart attacks and other CV disease.

However, this interpretation should be exercised with some caution and, despite the apparent success of the various trials, it is well recognized that sustaining lifestyle modifications in individual patients is often unsuccessful and thus, in the vast majority of cases, drug treatment in addition to lifestyle modification will be necessary to achieve good long-term blood pressure control.

The principles of drug treatment

Drug treatments may be given alone or in combination, but the ultimate aim is to control hypertension and normalize blood pressure without causing any symptomatic side-effects, adverse metabolic effects or long-term toxicity. The simplest drug regimen is preferred and, in this respect, to make it as easy as possible to adhere to treatment, most doctors prefer to use drugs which are effective when administered only once daily. Once-daily regimens can be considered preferable, and indeed do offer advantage by way of improved compliance. However, it should be recognized that although many antihypertensive agents are approved for once-daily administration, the same total daily dose given in a twice-daily dosing regimen may provide more appropriate blood pressure control by way of a smoother and more consistent antihypertensive effect.

The "older" drugs, thiazide diuretics and beta-blockers, are still widely recommended as first choice agents, but there is a current preference for individualized or "tailored" drug treatment, i.e. the selection of particular drug types (classes) because they are best suited to the particular requirements of the individual patient.

The response to the introduction of drug treatment is then evaluated over a period of weeks or months, with repeat blood pressure measurements. It may be necessary to increase the dosage if the effect is insufficient and if there are no side-effects; alternatively, if side-effects do occur, or if there is clearly no useful blood pressure response, then it is preferable to change to an alternative type of drug treatment. As a further alternative, however, combinations of two or more drugs may prove particularly suitable, not only for achieving "tight" blood pressure control, but also for "tailoring" treatment to match individual patient requirements.

First-line antihypertensive drugs

A wide range of suitable first-line antihypertensive drugs is now available and the classes of drugs currently in most widespread use are:

1. Thiazide diuretics.
2. Selective beta-adrenoceptor antagonists (beta-blockers).
3. Calcium channel blockers (CCBs)/calcium antagonists.
4. Angiotensin-converting enzyme inhibitors (ACEIs).
5. Angiotensin (AT1) receptor antagonists.

Appendix 1 provides a list of the most widely used antihypertensives, along with their trade names in the UK.

Thiazide diuretics

These drugs act on the kidney to increase sodium excretion and urine volume (Table 9); although this diuretic activity was initially thought to be the mechanism by which blood pressure was reduced, it is now recognized that the antihypertensive effect is not directly related to the diuretic potency but instead to other effects which cause subtle alterations (reductions) in the contractility of blood vessels. Thus, although thiazide-type diuretics are not powerful diuretics, they are the preferred types for the treatment of hypertension. The antihypertensive effect

Classification and site of action of diuretics

	Site of action	Comment
Thiazides		
Bendrofluazide Hydrochlorthiazide Chlorthalidone	Proximal part of the distal tubule	All have antihypertensive efficacy. Minor doubts regarding optimal dose range
Thiazide-like diuretics		
Indapamide	Proximal part of the distal tubule	Although indapamide was developed to produce a sulphonamide derivative that would dissociate thiazide-like antihypertensive effects from diuretic effects, there is little clinical evidence to suggest that it dffers substantially from thiazides
Loop diuretics		
Frusemide (furosemide) Bumetanide	Ascending limb of the loop of Henle	Potent diuretic and saliuretic, but less useful for treating hypertension
Potassium-sparing diuretics		
Bendrofluazide Amiloride	Distal tubule – adosterone antagonist Distal tubule – sodium– potassium exchange	May be particularly useful/effective when hyperaldosteronism is implicated. May cause hyperkalaemia in renal failure and the elderly

Table 9. Classification and site of action of diuretics.

of thiazide diuretics manifests at relatively low dosages (e.g. 2.5 mg bendrofluazide; 12.5 mg hydrochlorthiazide) and, in terms of blood pressure reduction, there is only a slight additional benefit from higher doses. A diuretic effect is observed on first dosing with the onset of the effect, usually observed within 1 hour and lasting for about 12 hours. With repeated dosing, the acute diuretic effect tends to diminish in the majority of hypertensive patients. The antihypertensive effect, however, is more gradual in onset and longer lasting, so that the blood pressure-lowering effect persists for more than 24 hours, and once-daily dosing is therefore appropriate.

Predictable adverse effects

Hypokalaemia

Because of the increased urinary loss of both sodium and potassium, there may be a reduction in blood potassium to levels below normal, although this is less likely with the low dosages currently preferred. Accordingly, it may be necessary to co-administer a potassium supplement or a potassium-sparing diuretic. If severe hypokalaemia persists during low-dose thiazide treatment, it should raise the suspicion of an underlying problem, such as mineralocorticoid excess, particularly hyperaldosteronism (Conn's syndrome).

Hyperuricaemia

Since thiazide diuretics also interfere with the excretion of uric acid, there may be an increased blood level of uric acid and, on occasion, the provocation of an acute gouty episode, particularly in the patient with some degree of renal impairment. This side-effect appears to be dose dependent and as such does not assume great importance with lower doses of diuretics.

Hyperglycaemia

Long-term diuretic therapy is associated with an impairment of glucose tolerance and an increased incidence of non-insulin-dependent (type II) diabetes mellitus. The mechanism appears to be mainly related to interference with the action of insulin in peripheral tissues (so-called "insulin resistance").

Hypercalcaemia
This is a rare adverse effect of thiazide diuretics resulting from reduced renal excretion of calcium.

Other adverse effects
Hyperlipidaemia
By mechanisms which are not entirely clear (although insulin resistance is again implicated), long-term use of thiazide diuretics is associated with changes in the plasma lipid profile with increases in total and low-density lipoprotein (LDL) cholesterol, and in total triglycerides, with a reduction in high-density lipoprotein (HDL) cholesterol.

Impotence/erectile dysfunction
This is a well-recognized but occasional problem with long-term diuretic treatment. The mechanism is unknown and the problem is usually reversible on treatment cessation.

Others
Thrombocytopenia and skin rash occur rarely. Thiazide diuretics, for example, bendrofluazide (2.5 mg daily), hydrochlorothiazide (12.5–25 mg daily) and chlorthalidone (12.5 or 25 mg daily), are widely used and are effective antihypertensive drugs in all severities of hypertension. Where the hypertension is complicated by chronic renal failure, or is proving refractory to treatment, it may be necessary to use a loop diuretic, such as furosemide (frusemide), torsemide or bumetanide. Since diuretic-induced hypokalaemia has been associated in the past with cardiac rhythm disturbances, it may be necessary to add a potassium-sparing drug such as amiloride or triamterene; in fact, the combination of a thiazide and a potassium-sparing drug has been shown in several clinical outcome trials to be a particularly effective first-line antihypertensive treatment. Although diuretic drugs are widely used as monotherapy, their effectiveness is also well established in combination with almost all other drug classes – for example, with a beta-blocker or an ACEI.

Beta-adrenoceptor antagonists (beta-blockers)

Beta-blockers antagonize the effects of both sympathetic nerve stimulation and circulating catecholamines such as noradrenaline and adrenaline. Beta-adrenoceptors are widely distributed throughout the body systems and are subclassified as beta-1- and beta-2-receptors. Beta-1-receptors predominate in the heart and beta-2-receptors predominate in other organs such as the lung, peripheral blood vessels and skeletal muscle.

1. Heart. Stimulation of beta-1-receptors in the sino-atrial node causes an increase in heart rate (a positive chronotropic effect) and stimulation of the beta-1-receptors in the myocardium increases the force of cardiac contractility (a positive inotropic effect).

2. Kidney. Stimulation of beta-receptors in the kidney promotes the release of renin from the juxtaglomerular cells and thereby increases the activity of the renin–angiotensin–aldosterone system.

3. Central and peripheral nervous system. Stimulation of beta-receptors in the brain stem and stimulation of pre-junctional beta-receptors in the periphery promote the release of neurotransmitters and increased sympathetic nervous system activity.

Overall, therefore, stimulation of beta-receptors in the heart, kidney and nervous system leads to an increase in cardiac output, an increase in peripheral vascular resistance, an increase in sympathetic nervous system activity and an increase in the activity of the renin–angiotensin–aldosterone system. Treatment with beta-blockers is able to antagonize all of these effects to cause a reduction in blood pressure, but it remains unclear which is the principal antihypertensive mechanism. Acutely, beta blockade leads to a reduction in cardiac output, but during long-term treatment the antihypertensive effect is instead associated with a reduction of the elevated peripheral vascular resistance.

All beta-blockers lower blood pressure to a similar extent, irrespective of their additional pharmacological characteristics. In hypertension, beta-1-selective ("cardioselective") drugs that can be administered once daily tend to be preferred (e.g.

bisoprolol, 10 mg daily). It is important to remember that, despite their apparent "cardioselectivity", these drugs are contraindicated in patients with asthma (see Table 10).

Predictable adverse effects
Bronchospasm
Beta-2-receptors mediate dilation of the bronchi; blockade of these receptors – which is a potential consequence of all currently available agents – may precipitate bronchospasm in susceptible individuals.

Bradycardia and impairment of myocardial contractility
An excessive reduction in heart rate and bradycardia are relatively common but seldom symptomatic. Rarely, an excessive reduction in inotropic activity may precipitate or exacerbate cardiac failure in a susceptible individual.

Classification of beta-blockers			
Clinical class	**Approved name**	**Beta-1 selectivity**	**Major route of elimination**
Non-selective	Propranolol	–	Liver
Selective	Atenolol	++	Kidney
	Bisoprolol	++	Liver/kidney
	Metoprolol	++	Liver
Additional properties			
Nitric oxide promotion	Nebivolol	+++	Liver
Intrinsic sympatho-mimetic activity (also partial agonist activity)	Pindolol	–	Liver
Anti-arrhythmic properties	Sotalol	–	Liver
Vasodilating mechanism	Carvedilol	–	Liver

Table 10. Classification of beta-blockers.

Peripheral vasoconstriction

The beta-2-receptors in the smooth muscle of peripheral arteries subserve a vasodilator role, especially in skeletal muscle beds, and blockade of these receptors leads to a relative vasoconstriction which typically gives rise to impairment of the peripheral circulation, leading to cold hands and feet and possibly the development of Raynaud's phenomenon or the worsening of pre-existing peripheral vascular disease.

CNS effects

Blockade of these beta-receptors is associated with reduced sympathetic outflow, which is the probable cause of a sense of malaise that may occur insidiously during long-term treatment. Vivid dreams, nightmares and, rarely, hallucinations may occur with highly lipid-soluble beta-blockers (propranolol in particular) because of their greater penetration into the CNS.

Tiredness and fatigue

Stimulation of beta-2-receptors in skeletal muscle is associated with increased muscle activity, and blockade of these receptors leads to a sense of tiredness and ready fatigue during exercise.

Masking of hypoglycaemia

The awareness of hypoglycaemia in the insulin-dependent diabetic depends partly upon sympathetic nervous activation. This response will be blunted by beta-blockers. This seems to be a theoretical rather than a practical issue in the great majority of patients.

Metabolic disturbances

Beta-blockers, especially non-selective agents, tend to increase triglycerides and reduce HDL cholesterol. They also interfere with peripheral insulin responsiveness, leading to relative insulin resistance. The mechanisms underlying these metabolic effects are unknown.

For all practical purposes, all of the beta-blockers are as effective as each other in reducing blood pressure; however, there are important pharmacological differences between the different agents.

Cardioselectivity
Some beta-blockers are considered to be non-selective in that they block both beta-1- and beta-2-receptors to a similar extent (e.g. propranolol, otimolol). The cardioselective agents (e.g. atenolol, metoprolol, bisoprolol) block beta-1-receptors to a greater extent than beta-2-receptors. However, selectivity is a relative term and it is important to recognize that, irrespective of their apparent "cardioselectivity", these drugs are contraindicated in people with asthma.

Intrinsic sympathomimetic activity
Like many competitive inhibitors, some beta-blockers stimulate the beta-receptors as well as block them, particularly when endogenous catecholamine levels are low. This intrinsic sympathomimetic activity or partial agonist activity is seen with pindolol and oxprenolol, and these agents may be less susceptible to producing bradycardia, but may possibly be less effective in their antihypertensive activity.

Lipophilicity
Some beta-blockers are much more lipophilic (lipid soluble) than others. Lipophilic compounds, because of their lipid-soluble nature, are more likely to enter the brain and cause central side-effects (e.g. propranolol). In contrast, hydrophilic (water-soluble) drugs (atenolol, nadolol) should cause less central side-effects. The different agents also differ in their excretion mechanisms, which may be an important determinant for drug selection when renal or hepatic impairment is present. Thus, lipophilic drugs are mainly eliminated by liver metabolism, whilst hydrophilic drugs are largely excreted unchanged by the kidneys.

Vasodilating beta-blockers
Some beta-blocking drugs have additional pharmacological properties which promote vasodilation (e.g. labetalol, which is a combined beta- and alpha-blocker, or carvedilol). There is no evidence that this dual action provides any overall advantage in terms either of improved outcome or reduced adverse effects.

Overall, it appears that, irrespective of their additional pharmacological characteristics, beta-blockers lower blood pressure to a similar extent. In hypertension, those which are beta-1 selective ("cardioselective"), and with genuine long duration of action such that they can be administered once daily, should be preferred (e.g. bisoprolol, 10 mg daily).

Calcium channel blockers/calcium antagonists

Mechanism of action

The increased peripheral vascular resistance of essential hypertension depends upon increased constrictor "tone" in peripheral blood vessels, which in turn reflects increased contractility of vascular smooth muscle. This process is calcium dependent and, fundamentally, all calcium antagonist drugs or calcium channel blockers (CCBs) are able to promote vasodilator activity by reducing calcium influx into the cell.

Intracellular calcium influx is also important in cardiac muscle, cardiac conducting tissue and the smooth muscle of the gastrointestinal tract; thus, the potential cardiac effects of calcium channel blockade are negative inotropic (reduced contractility), chronotropic (reduced heart rate) and dromotropic activity (slowed conduction of the cardiac impulse), whereas the gastrointestinal effects lead to constipation. These effects vary with different agents according to their different abilities to penetrate cardiac and other tissues and, in particular, because the receptor or recognition site close to the calcium channel is slightly different for each drug class.

Thus, although they are often referred to as a single class, there are very clear distinctions to be made between the three principal types of calcium antagonist drug:

1. Dihydropyridine derivatives – prototype drug, nifedipine.
2. Phenylalkalamines – prototype drug, verapamil.
3. Benzothiazipine derivatives – prototype drug, diltiazem.

The principal differences between these three main classes are that the dihydropyridine derivatives have pronounced peripheral vasodilator properties and minimal direct cardiac effects, whereas verapamil and diltiazem have significant cardiac effects whereby they are often described as "rate-limiting" agents, i.e. they have a bradycardic effect.

Pharmacologically predictable adverse effects

- Dihydropyridines.
    — Short or intermediate-acting agents: there is a well-recognized pattern of "vasodilator" side-effects with headache and facial flushing and an associated reflex activation of the sympathetic nervous system, which provokes tachycardia and palpitations. These symptoms usually decline with time.
    — Long(er)-acting agents: the longer-acting agents and the longer-acting formulations, however, are less likely to promote so-called "vasodilator" effects. However, swelling of the ankles is a well-recognized long-term effect, especially in women. This is not attributable to a generalized fluid retention (and therefore does not usually respond to diuretic treatment) but, instead, reflects a drug-related disturbance of the haemodynamics of the microcirculation in the periphery, plus the effect of gravity.
- Verapamil. The early-onset vasodilator effects are less common with verapamil but the cardiac effects may manifest as bradycardia or atrioventricular conduction delay. Constipation is a well-recognized symptomatic complaint.
- Diltiazem. Early vasodilator effects are again less apparent, but bradycardia and atrioventricular conduction effects are recognized. Skin rash occurs occasionally.

All types of calcium antagonist drugs are effective antihypertensive agents because of their peripheral vasodilator activity (Table 11). The long-acting dihydropyridine drugs are more widely used in hypertension because of their lack of negative cardiac effects and because of their suitability for once-daily dosing. Such long duration of action may be achieved by drugs with differing characteristics. There is no doubt that amlodipine offers a long duration of action, which has proven advantage in the setting of sub-optimal compliance and this directly associated with its long elimination half-life.

In contrast, the nifedipine gastrointestinal therapeutic system (GITS) relies upon a sophisticated formulation to provide a broadly similar long-acting, once-daily drug. More recently, a series of lipophilic dihydropyridine calcium antagonists have been developed (lacidipine, lercanidipine). These agents, despite having a relatively short half-life, have been shown to be suitable for once-daily administration due to their long-lasting affinity for the binding sites at a tissue level.

The use of dihydropyridine calcium antagonists may also offer an advantage in the practical implication that, when drug combination is required, a dihydropyridine CCB in combination with a beta-blocker is a preferred and effective combination in both hypertension and angina, whilst the negative effects of

Characteristics of calcium antagonists

	Plasma half-life (hours)	Frequency of administration
Dihydropyridine derivatives		
• **Short-acting**		
Nifedipine	4–6	Multiple times/day
Nicardipine	4–6	Multiple times/day
• **Intermediate**		
Isradipine	8–12	Once or twice daily
Lacidipine	6–8	Once daily
Lercanidipine	6–10	Once daily
Felodipine ER	2–9	Once daily
• **Long-acting**		
Amlodipine	>40	Once daily
Nifedipine GITS	Formulation dependent	Once daily
Phenylalkylamine		
Verapamil	10–12	Multiple times/day*
Benzothiazepine		
Diltiazem	8–10	Multiple times/day*

*Some modified release formulations are suitable for once/twice daily dosing.

Table 11. Characteristics of calcium antagonists.

the beta-blocker on cardiac performance are additive to those of verapamil and diltiazam. Furthermore, combining beta-blockers with the non-dihydropyridine calcium antagonists may lead to clinically significant bradycardia or atrioventricular conduction abnormalities.

Angiotensin-converting enzyme inhibitors

Mechanism of action

Angiotensin-converting enzyme inhibitors (ACEIs) are drugs which competitively inhibit the activity of angiotensin-converting enzyme (ACE; also termed kininase II) to prevent the formation of angiotensin II from its inactive precursor, angiotensin I (Figure 28). Angiotensin II has a range of activities but, most importantly, it is a potent vasoconstrictor, it promotes aldosterone release and it facilitates the activity of the sympathetic nervous system both centrally and peripherally. Whilst the reduction in blood pressure following ACE inhibition is greatest in patients with a stimulated renin–angiotensin system (such as occurs in sodium depletion, or with diuretic treatment, or in renal artery stenosis or in malignant phase hypertension), it is now recognized that ACEIs also lower blood pressure in essential hypertensive patients with normal or low

The renin-angiotensin system

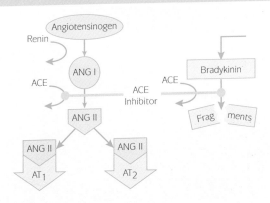

Figure 28. The renin–angiotensin system: ACE inhibition.

activity of the renin–angiotensin system. Although these drugs can functionally be considered to be peripheral vasodilators, it is noteworthy that the response to ACEIs does not provoke any reflex tachycardia.

There are some important pharmacological differences among ACEIs. For example, the prototype drug captopril is rapidly absorbed but has a short duration of action and is usually administered twice or three times daily. Enalapril, like the majority of the later ACEIs, is an inactive prodrug which needs to be hydrolysed in the liver to its active form enalaprilat. Lisinopril is an analogue of enalapril and is itself active without conversion.

Predictable adverse effects
Profound hypotension
This may complicate the first dose of an ACEI drug, especially in patients with heart failure who have marked sodium or volume depletion and in whom the renin–angiotensin system is activated. Severe hypotension only rarely occurs in uncomplicated essential hypertension.

Impairment of renal function
This is a recognized complication of ACEI treatment, particularly in patients with renovascular disease (particularly bilateral renal artery stenosis) in whom reversible (usually) renal failure may be precipitated.

Cough
This is the most frequent adverse effect and is probably attributable to the effect on the kinin system, rather than upon ACE inhibition itself. ACE, as a biochemical entity, is alternatively known as kininase II; as such, it is responsible for the breakdown of kinins, which have vasodilator and other properties. Inhibition of kininase II leads to accumulation of kinins, which promote vasodilator activity (and contribute to the overall haemodynamic effectiveness of ACEIs). However, kinin accumulation "sensitizes" the airways; thus, non-productive, irritant cough is widely reported in the treatment

of hypertension in up to about 15% of patients. The reported incidence is considerably less in patients with cardiac failure, presumably as a reflection of their higher background incidences of respiratory symptoms.

Hyperkalaemia

Increases in serum potassium and, occasionally, hyperkalaemia (serum potassium > 5.5 mmol/l) occur because ACEIs have potassium-sparing effects (mediated via the reduction in aldosterone). Hyperkalaemia may also complicate ACEI treatment if a potassium-sparing diuretic is used, or if the patient is receiving NSAIDs; both of these potential complications are particularly likely if renal impairment is also present.

Other adverse effects

Angio-oedema is a rare but well-recognized class effect which has also been attributed to kinin potentiation.

Although the majority of these agents are recommended for once-daily dosing, with many it appears that a more consistent response is produced by twice-daily administration. In elderly patients, or in patients with compromised renal function, or in patients with cardiac failure, it is advisable to initiate treatment with lower than usual dosages.

In general, these drugs are considered to be well tolerated by patients, especially in comparison with "old-fashioned" agents such as sympatholytic drugs. ACEI drugs combine well with thiazide diuretics, and with calcium antagonists, to produce overall antihypertensive effects which are at least additive. However, it is recommended that potassium supplements and potassium-sparing diuretics should not be used in combination because hyperkalaemia may result, especially if there is pre-existing renal impairment.

In contrast, the effectiveness of ACEIs in both hypertension and cardiac failure may be compromised by NSAIDs which, if possible, should be avoided. One exception to this may be celecoxib, a COX-2-specific inhibitor which appears to be well tolerated when used in hypertensive patients controlled with ACEIs.[41]

Angiotensin (AT₁) receptor antagonists

Mechanism of action

This relatively new class of drugs acts via the renin–angiotensin system by directly blocking the action of angiotensin II at the angiotensin II receptor (AT$_1$ subtype; Figure 29). Blockade of the AT$_1$ receptor results in increased local and, to an extent, circulating levels of angiotensin II. This may provide an additional indirect mechanism of action in that the increased angiotensin II may act directly on the AT$_2$ receptor, producing beneficial effects that complement the selective blockade of the AT$_1$ receptor. All of the widely available angiotensin receptor blockers (losartan, irbesartan, valsartan, candesartan, telmisartan, eprosartan and omesartan) are highly selective antagonists at the AT$_1$ receptor. There are differences in receptor blockade, which are usually described as "insurmountable" or "partially insurmountable". These differences are apparent in *in vitro* experiments in which the antagonist is introduced into the system prior to the addition of the agonist; thus, the clinical relevance, if any, of the different binding characteristics remains to be elucidated. Differences are also apparent in the disposition characteristics of the different drugs, but again the clinical

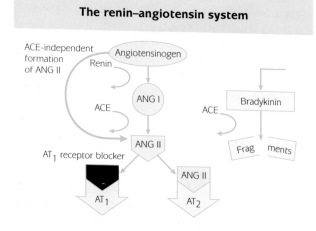

The renin–angiotensin system

ACE-independent formation of ANG II

Renin

Angiotensinogen

ANG I

ACE

ACE

Bradykinin

ANG II

Frag ments

AT$_1$ receptor blocker

ANG II

AT$_1$

AT$_2$

Figure 29. The renin–angiotensin system: selective angiotensin receptor (AT$_1$) blockade.

relevance of these differences remains unclear. However, unlike all the other currently available agents, losartan largely depends upon the generation of an active metabolite EXP3174 for its antihypertensive effect. The parent drug, losartan, also has the unique property of being uricosuric, a property which is independent of its action at the AT_1 receptor. The clinical relevance of the reductions in uric acid observed during long-term therapy remain to be elucidated, but uric acid is re-emerging as an independent risk factor for CVD.

The clinical indications, overall efficacy and potential adverse effects of this class are similar to those of the ACEIs, but with one notable difference – the absence of cough (and angio-oedema) as an adverse effect (Table 9). Angiotensin antagonist drugs act specifically to block angiotensin II receptors and unlike ACEIs they have no effect on the kinin system, which may well account for the absence of cough. It may also be associated with a reduced incidence of angio-oedema when compared to ACEIs.

In general, the antihypertensive effects of these agents are equivalent to those of ACEIs, but the major advantage of these drugs is that they are very well tolerated with no class-specific adverse effects and placebo-like tolerability. This undoubtedly offers an advantage which is apparent in persistence rates, such that after 1 and 4 years treatment, more patients are sustained on their initially prescribed angiotensin antagonist than any other class of antihypertensive agent (Figure 30).[42] A number of randomized outcome trials have recently been reported and whilst these are discussed further in a later section of this chapter (Recent clinical outcome trials), the evidence indicates that they are able to significantly reduce CV morbidity and mortality in specific groups of hypertensive patients.

Alternative antihypertensive drugs

These first five drug classes dominate current clinical practice: this is a function of established effectiveness, outcome evidence and familiarity. Other agents, especially those with alternative attributes – fewer adverse effects or potentially beneficial ancillary properties – constitute important alternative treatments.

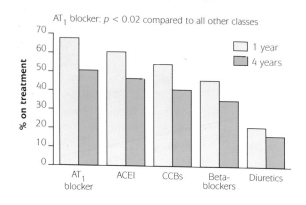

Figure 30. The persistence with the initially prescribed agent after 1 and 4 years treatment with all the major classes of antihypertensives. Data from reference 42.

Selective alpha-1-adrenoceptor antagonists (alpha-blockers)

These drugs act via selective blockade of peripheral alpha-1-adrenoceptors to produce their vasodilator effects, but they are not widely used first-line agents. Instead, they tend to be reserved for use as a combination or "add-on" treatment, particularly for patients in whom there is a concomitant problem, such as benign prostatic enlargement, type II diabetes or dyslipidaemia. Alpha-1-adrenoceptor antagonists are the only agents which, in addition to blood pressure reduction, cause modest improvements in the blood lipid profile with reductions in total cholesterol, LDL cholesterol and total triglycerides, and an increase in HDL cholesterol.

In the past, alpha-blockers have been associated with a pronounced "first-dose" hypotensive side-effect which constitutes a postural hypotensive response after the initial dosage, accompanied by reflex tachycardia and a sense of palpitations. This first-dose effect was particularly associated with short-acting agents, particularly prazosin, and is much less problematical with longer-acting agents, such as doxazosin, particularly in its new, modified-release formulation.

Recently, the arm of the ALLHAT study comparing doxazosin with chlorthalidone was terminated early on the grounds of an apparent increase in risk of developing heart failure with doxazosin and, more importantly, the likely inability of the trial to demonstrate superiority for CV outcomes with the alpha-blocker when compared to the diuretic, were the trial have run to completion.[43] The finding of an apparent increase in risk of heart failure associated with doxazosin should be interpreted with some caution. The information collected on the clinical status of the patients prior to entering the trial was very limited and in addition the trial was based upon comparing monotherapy with the two agents. Given that the use of doxazosin is predominantly associated with add-on combination therapy, extrapolation from the ALLHAT trial is inappropriate, although a recent analysis and publication in the *Annals of Internal Medicine* showed that combination therapy with doxazosin in ALLHAT still had an increased stroke and CV event rate compared to diuretic-based combination groups.

Centrally acting agents

Agents acting on alpha-2-adrenoceptors, or related receptors in the brain stem, are known to reduce sympathetic outflow and lead to a reduction in blood pressure. These agents act upon regulatory and inhibitory neurotransmitter systems within the CNS but, generally, they have been insufficiently selective or specific to avoid unwanted symptomatic adverse CNS effects.

Thus, centrally acting agents (e.g. clonidine and alpha-methylodopa) are no longer widely used because of their poor side-effect profiles (particularly the CNS depressant effects) and because of the development of newer comparably effective alternative agents. However, alpha-methyldopa is still used to treat hypertension in pregnancy, especially where hypertension precedes pregnancy or is identified in the first or middle trimester. This is justified by the long-term experience of foetal and maternal safety.

Moxonidine development was discontinued in the USA in 1999 or 2000 due to sedating side-effects, increased motor vehicle accidents, etc.

Drugs with vasodilator properties

Drugs with overt vasodilator activity have been widely used in the past, particularly in combination with beta-blockers and diuretics. Such "triple therapy" proved particularly effective because the beta-blocker and diuretic attenuated the reflex activation of the sympathetic and renin–angiotensin–aldosterone systems which, typically, was provoked with these agents. Direct acting vasodilators, such as hydralazine and minoxidil, are particularly likely to provoke reflex tachycardia and fluid retention, and their vasodilator action was also associated with symptomatic adverse effects such as facial flushing and headache.

Recent clinical outcome trials

As discussed in earlier sections of this book, the benefits of treating mild to moderate (Stage I to III) hypertension were established in a series of placebo-controlled trials whose results were definitively summarized in a subsequent meta-analysis. The more recent clinical outcome trials in hypertension have focused attention on high-risk patients: on patients with hypertension and diabetes; on the elderly hypertensive and on ISH; and on the effectiveness of some of the newer classes of antihypertensive agent (i.e. CCBs, ACEI drugs and angiotensin receptor antagonists rather than thiazide diuretics and beta-blocker drugs).

The Syst-Eur study

The Syst-Eur study was the first intervention trial, with appropriate randomization, to show that an antihypertensive treatment regimen based upon a CCB provided protection against CV morbidity and mortality.[44] This was essentially the last of the placebo-controlled, double-blind trials targeting the treatment of ISH in the elderly. The trial was terminated early on ethical grounds as it was apparent that the benefits were substantial. This was characterized by statistically significant reductions in all CV end-points and in fatal and non-fatal stroke. There also was a reduction in MI but this did not achieve statistical significance, probably as a consequence of the early termination of the trial. It is noteworthy that in similar patient populations, albeit with different treatment regimens, the outcomes in the SHEP and Syst-Eur studies showed a high degree of commonality (Table 12). In SHEP, monotherapy predominated; only about 20% of patients were on atenolol or reserpine.

The HOT study

The HOT study differed from all other randomized hypertension trials in that it did not compare different classes of antihypertensive agents.[34] Instead, it aimed at assessing the optimal diastolic blood pressure in the treatment of

Isolated systolic hypertension in the elderly: comparison of Syst-Eur and SHEP		
	Syst-Eur	**SHEP**
Drug use		
First line	Nitrendipine (84%)	Chlorthalidone (69%)
Second line	Enalapril (33%)	Atenolol (23%)
Third line	HCTZ (16%)	Reserpine (23%)
BP response (mmHg)	10/5	12/4
Relative risk reduction (%)		
Stroke	42**	36**
MI	30	27*
CV events	31**	32**
All-cause mortality	14	13
Absolute benefit[†]		
Stroke	34	33
CV events	19	17

*$p < 0.05$; **$p < 0.01$.
[†]Number of patients to treat for 5 years to prevent one event.

Table 12. Isolated systolic hypertension in the elderly: comparison of Syst-Eur and SHEP.

hypertension. Nearly 19,000 patients were randomized to achieve one of three target diastolic blood pressures: ≤ 90, ≤ 85 and ≤ 80 mmHg. Felodipine (modified release) was used as the initial therapy, with the addition of other agents according to a five-step regimen. Whilst 92% of patients achieved diastolic blood pressure levels of ≤ 90 mmHg (from an initial mean level of 105 mmHg), achieving the lower target pressures proved to be more difficult and ultimately the mean values in the three groups were 85, 83 and 81 mmHg respectively. Despite this similarity in achieved blood pressure, all major CV events (fatal and non-fatal stroke, MI, CV mortality) showed a progressive decline in relation to the target blood pressure category and this trend was significant for fatal and non-fatal MI. In relation to the achieved diastolic blood pressure, the lowest incidence of all major CV events combined was found to be 83 mmHg. The overall trends in the study as a whole were even more apparent in the subgroup analysis of diabetic patients, in whom there was a statistically significant relationship between lower randomized blood pressure (Figure 31) and a lower incidence of CV events.

UKPDS

When compared to the HOT study, the UKPDS study was a much smaller study in 1148 hypertensives with type II diabetes but with a longer follow-up period of 8 years.[45] Patients were randomized to "tight" or "less tight" blood pressure control and the average difference achieved at the end of the trial between the two groups was 10/5 mmHg. Tight blood pressure control resulted in a number of statistically significant benefits with regard to macro- and microvascular events (Figure 32). Thus, as in the HOT study diabetic subgroup, the benefits of "aggressive" lowering of blood pressure were clearly demonstrated in these high-risk patients. The investigators also sought to discriminate between the different treatment regimens, but failed to show any significant differences between those based upon the beta-blocker atenolol and the ACEI captopril. However, the power of the study to discriminate any possible significant difference was very low.

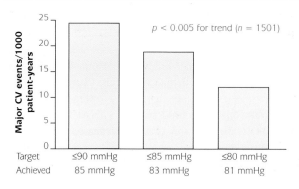

Figure 31. The decrease in cardiovascular risk in diabetic patients randomized to three different target pressures in the HOT study. Data from reference 35.

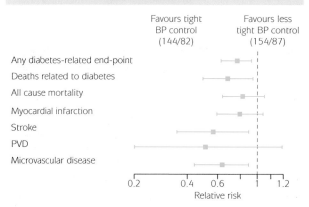

Figure 32. The UKPDS study: benefits of tight blood pressure control in type II diabetes. Data from reference 45.

The CAPPP study

Despite ACEI drugs having been widely available for over 15 years, the CAPPP study was the first intervention trial in hypertension to compare treatment based on an ACEI with treatment based on diuretics and/or beta-blockers.[46] Over 11,000 hypertensive patients were studied in a prospective, randomized, open, blinded end-point evaluation (PROBE) trial conducted in Scandinavia. Overall, none of the primary CV end-points differed between the two groups and, as with many other trials, a substantial number of patients were receiving combination therapies in both arms of the study.

The STOP Hypertension-2 study

The STOP Hypertension-2 study compared conventional antihypertensive drugs (atenolol, metoprolol, pindolol, or hydrochlorothiazide plus amiloride) with newer drugs (enalapril, lisinopril, felodipine or isradipine) in a prospective randomized trial in 6614 patients aged 70–84 years.[47] Equivalent blood pressure reductions were observed in all treatment groups. The primary combined end-point of fatal stroke, fatal MI and other fatal CVD occurred at similar rates in the conventional drugs group and in the newer drugs group (Figure 33). The secondary end-points similarly showed no differences between the two treatment groups, and it was judged that old and new antihypertensive drugs were similar in their abilities to reduce CV mortality and major CV events and that decreasing blood pressure was the most important factor in prevention of these events.

INSIGHT

The INSIGHT study was a prospective double-blind trial in over 6000 high-risk hypertensive patients aged 55–80 years.[48] The patients were randomly assigned to treatment with either nifedipine (30 mg) in a long-acting formulation (GITS) or co-amilozide (25 mg hydrochlorthiazide plus 2.5 mg amiloride). Blood pressure control was equivalent in each group and the two treatment modalities were equally effective in preventing CV complications (stroke, MI, CHF, CV deaths).

The NORDIL study

The NORDIL study was very similar in design to the CAPPP study and it compared the effects on outcome of a diltiazem-based regimen with that of a conventional regimen based on diuretics and/or beta-blockers.[49] Nearly 11,000 hypertensive patients aged 50–74 years were randomized to one or other of the two treatment regimens. No difference was apparent between the different arms of the study with respect to the primary end-point (fatal and non-fatal stroke, MI, plus other CV mortality) with a relative risk (RR) between the two groups of 1.00 (95% CI: 0.87–1.15). The secondary end-point of fatal and non-fatal stroke showed a statistically significant benefit for the CCB-based regimen (RR = 0.80; 95% CI: 0.65–0.99). At the conclusion of the trial, only 50% of patients in the CCB arm and 45% of those in the "conventional" therapy arm remained on their randomized therapy. This again illustrates that combined antihypertensive therapy is required in large proportions of patients to achieve target blood pressure.

The HOPE study

The HOPE study was not strictly targeted at hypertensive patients, but it warrants consideration in that it provides further information on the potential benefits of ACE inhibition in high-risk patients.[36]

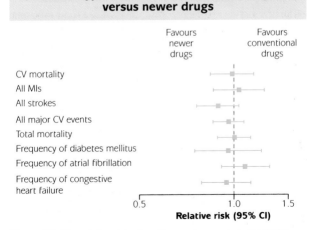

Figure 33. The relative risk of cardiovascular events in the STOP Hypertension-2 trial: comparison of conventional and newer drugs. Data from reference 47.

The trial involved older patients who had a high risk of CV events but who did not have left ventricular dysfunction or heart failure. The study assessed the addition in a randomized blinded fashion of ramipril or placebo to existing "standard" therapy (just under 50% were receiving antihypertensive drugs for existing high blood pressure). At the conclusion of the study, it was apparent that ACEI treatment significantly reduced rates of mortality, MI, stroke and heart failure in these high-risk patients (Figure 34). Since the mean blood pressure differences between the two groups was 3/2 mmHg, the investigators concluded that the benefits were unlikely to be solely due to blood pressure-lowering effects. They justified this by predicting the benefit that might have been accrued from the blood pressure difference based both on the outcomes in the placebo group in the trial and predicted from a meta-analysis of all trials. On this basis, the observed benefit from ramipril was much greater than that from the blood pressure reduction alone (Table 13). However, this apparently small difference in blood pressure should still be interpreted with some caution. Firstly, blood pressure assessments were made on a somewhat *ad hoc* basis using recordings in the clinic at times which were not specified, and the ramipril was dosed in the evening; additionally, and perhaps of considerable importance, much more substantial differences in blood pressure were apparent in a small subgroup of patients who undertook ambulatory BP recordings. It is important to bear in mind that the importance of small differences in blood pressure in high-risk populations should not be underestimated – for example, a 50% reduction in CV events was apparent in the diabetic subgroup in the HOT study with a difference in achieved diastolic blood pressure of only 4 mmHg.

Recent meta-analyses

Whilst recent trials have advanced the knowledge base necessary for appropriate treatment of hypertension, none in isolation can be considered to be definitive. As described earlier, the technique of meta-analysis has been usefully applied to define the benefits of treatment of mild to moderate hypertension. The technique has also been applied to address the question "what constitutes the best first choice of antihypertensive therapy?"

Two such meta-analyses have recently been performed.[50,51] Both essentially addressed the same issue as to whether the newer agents – calcium antagonists and ACEIs – were as effective, better than, or less effective than conventional therapies. There were subtle, but potentially important,

Estimates of blood pressure contribution to the benefits observed in HOPE

	Risk reduction (%)	
	Myocardial infaction	**Stroke**
Observed reduction in ramipril group	20	32
Predicted reduction based on BP reduction		
Corrected using meta-analysis data	5	13
Correction based on placebo group	5.5	7

Table 13. Estimates of blood pressure contribution to the benefits observed in HOPE.

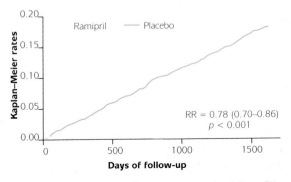

Figure 34. The HOPE study: primary outcome – death from CV causes, myocardial infarction and stroke. Data from reference 36

differences between the publications with regard to the trials that were incorporated in the meta-analyses but, overall, the summarizing results did not show major differences. The main area of contention related to the comparison of CCBs and other drugs. The summarizing findings are presented in Figures 35 and 36, and the relative consistency between the two studies is immediately apparent. In both interpretations CCBs fared less well with respect to coronary artery disease, congestive heart failure and major CV events, which attained statistical significance in one analysis but not in the other. By way of contrast, the opposite was true for stroke, where the incidence was reduced by CCBs compared to other agents in both studies, but only achieved statistical significance in one of the analyses. Overall, the findings of the two studies are consistent with each other and they both provide strong evidence of the benefits of antihypertensive treatment based on ACEIs and CCBs. However, the evidence for differences in outcome between different treatment regimens was relatively weak.

Trials of angiotensin receptor antagonists in type II diabetes

Results defining the role of angiotensin receptor antagonists in the management of type II diabetes were recently reported in three different studies.

The RENAAL study was performed in type II diabetic patients with established nephropathy who were randomized to either standard care or losartan in addition to the standard care.[52] The composite end-point of time to first, doubling of serum creatinine, ESRD or death was significantly reduced by 16% in patients randomized to losartan (Figure 37). As with many other studies in high-risk patients, combination therapy was required in the vast majority of patients and, overall, approximately four drugs were required in each patient to achieve blood pressure control.

The second angiotensin receptor antagonist study, the IDNT study, was similar to RENAAL but in this instance included not only the angiotensin receptor antagonist irbesartan and placebo, but also the calcium antagonist amlodipine by way of an active control.[53] The primary composite end-point was

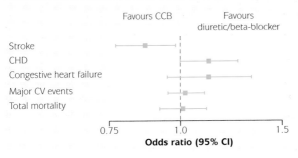

Figure 35. The meta-analysis of trial in hypertension: calcium antagonists compared with other agents. Data from reference 50.

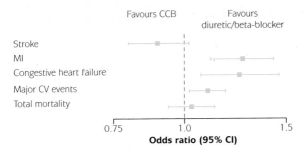

Figure 36. Meta-analysis of trials in hypertension: calcium antagonists compared with other agents. Data from reference 51.

similar to that in RENAAL and again the greatest benefit with respect to a reno-protective effect was associated with the angiotensin receptor antagonist, despite equivalent blood pressure control to that achieved with amlodipine (Figure 38). However, CV end-points did not differ between the irbesartan and amlodipine arms of the trial.

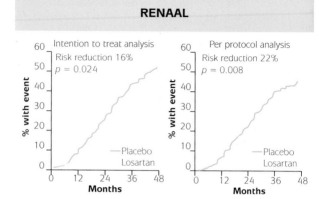

Figure 37. The primary end-point results of the RENAAL trial. Data from 52.

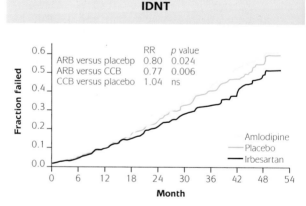

Figure 38. The primary end-point results of the IDNT trial. Data from reference 53.

Finally, the IRMA 2 trial addressed the issue as to whether angiotensin receptor blockade could effectively delay the development of diabetic nephropathy in type II diabetics.[54] At the conclusion of the trial, treatment with irbesartan when compared to placebo was associated with a 70% reduction in progression to nephropathy, a 54% reduction in urinary albumin excretion and a 1.7-fold greater regression to normoalbuminuria. These benefits were particularly apparent for the higher daily dose of 300 mg irbesartan compared to the lower dose of 150 mg.

These three studies have demonstrated the benefits of angiotensin receptor blockade in the treatment of type II diabetes, with the overall conclusion that the reno-protective effects were greater than that anticipated from blood pressure control alone.

LIFE

The most recently published trial in high-risk hypertensive patients is the LIFE trial, in which over 9000 hypertensives with established left ventricular hypertrophy (aged 55–80 years) were randomly assigned to treatment with losartan or atenolol, to which hydrochlorthiazide and other agents could be added where blood pressure control was not achieved.[55] At the end of the follow-up period (mean 4.7 years), the achieved systolic blood pressure was 1.3 mmHg lower and diastolic blood pressure was 0.4 mmHg higher in the losartan group compared to the atenolol group. The primary composite end-point (CV mortality, fatal/non-fatal stroke and fatal/non-fatal MI) was reduced by 14.6% (p < 0.009) in the losartan arm compared to the atenolol arm (Figure 39). When

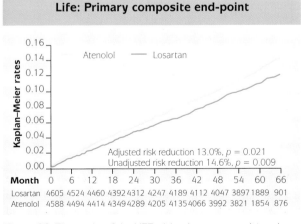

Figure 39. The results of the LIFE trial: primary composite end-point. Data from reference 55.

adjustment was made for Framingham risk score and ECG left ventricular hypertrophy at baseline, the risk reduction was 13.0% (p < 0.021). The benefits associated with angiotensin receptor blockade were predominantly associated with a 25% reduction in stroke (Table 14) and indeed there was a small but statistically non-significant increase in MI in the losartan group compared to atenolol. Losartan, which was significantly better tolerated than atenolol, was also shown to reduce the rate of new onset of diabetes and protect against CV events in diabetics.

ALLHAT and the 2nd Australian National Blood Pressure Study Group

The final results of the ALLHAT trial demonstrated that for the formal primary endpoint of fatal coronary heart disease and nonfatal myocardial infarction, there were no meaningful differences among the 3 remaining treatment groups.[56] The study event rate for chlorthalidone was 11.5%, with minimally lower point estimates for lisinopril (11.4%) and amlodipine (11.3%) (Figure 40). This occurred despite the fact that the systolic blood pressure was not as well controlled in the lisinopril and amlodipine groups as in the diuretic group (Figure 41)

End-points in LIFE trial – intention to treat analysis

	Losartan (n = 4605)	Atenolol (n = 4588)	Unadjusted RR (%)	p	Adjusted RR (%)	p
1° composite	508	588	−15	0.009	−13	0.021
CV mortality	204	234	−13	0.14	−11	0.21
Stroke	232	309	−26	0.0006	−25	0.001
MI	198	188	+5	0.63	+7	0.49
Total mortality	383	431	−12	0.08	−10	0.13
New onset DM	241	319	−25	<0.001	−25	<0.001

Table 14. End-points in LIFE trial – intention to treat analysis.

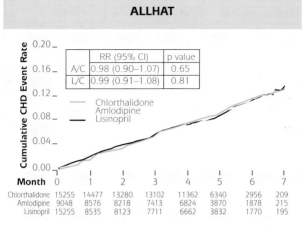

Figure 40. The time to event of the primary endpoint of fatal coronary heart disease and nonfatal MI according to the 3 treatment groups of diuretic, ACE inhibitor, and calcium antagonist in the ALLHAT trial.

Secondary endpoints in ALLHAT included prevention of stroke and development of congestive heart failure. The most notable difference in ALLHAT were the stroke rates: compared with the diuretic, the stroke event rate during treatment with amlodipine was 7% lower (not statistically significant) and was observed in nearly all of the subgroups in ALLHAT. Chlorthalidone reduced the stroke event rate by 15% when compared to the ACE inhibitor lisinopril (statistically significant, $p < 0.05$). Of note, the stroke rates for white patients were nearly identical on the diuretic and ACE inhibitor whereas for the African-American population, there was a highly significant ($p < 0.001$) reduction in stroke rate by 40% on the diuretic compared to the ACE inhibitor (Figure 42). This is not surprising as there was a 4 mmHg disparity in systolic BP reduction on the ACE inhibitor compared to the diuretic; this difference could explain much if not all of the stroke excess in the higher risk African-American patient population.

Finally, the results of the ALLHAT trial suggested that the diuretic was superior to both the ACE inhibitor lisinopril and the

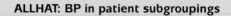

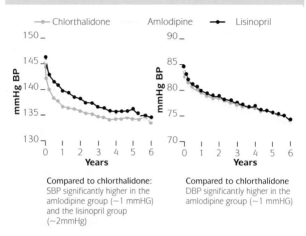

ALLHAT: BP in patient subgroupings

Compared to chlorthalidone:
SBP significantly higher in the amlodipine group (~1 mmHG) and the lisinopril group (~2mmHg)

Compared to chlorthalidone
DBP significantly higher in the amlodipine group (~1 mmHG)

Figure 41. Blood pressure values during the 7 year period of treatment in the 3 treatment groups in ALLHAT.

calcium antagonist amlodipine in the prevention of heart failure. The absolute differences in cumulative hospitalised and non-hospitalised heart failure rates were approximately 1% less on the diuretic compared to the calcium antagonist group and 0.6% less on the ACE inhibitor. There are problems with this assessment however, since none of these patients had a careful diagnosis of congestive heart failure and this particular endpoint was not formally evaluated by an endpoints committee. Furthermore, it was noted that the onset of heart failure occurred quite rapidly after randomisation leading some experts to believe that patients developing heart failure soon after entering the trial were actually unsuspected heart failure patients who simply became fluid-overloaded when their prior therapy of diuretics was discontinued.

To make matters more complex, the 2nd Australian National Blood Pressure Study Group recently reported conflicting final results of this 6083 patient trial which utilized either a thiazide diuretic (typically hydrochlorothiazide) or an ACE inhibitor (typically enalapril).[57] The primary endpoint of cardiovascular events and unexplained death was reduced significantly by the

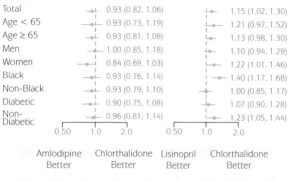

ALLHAT: Relative risk of stroke according to patient subgroupings

	Amlodipine / Chlorthalidone	Lisinopril / Chlorthalidone
Total	0.93 (0.82, 1.06)	1.15 (1.02, 1.30)
Age < 65	0.93 (0.73, 1.19)	1.21 (0.97, 1.52)
Age ≥ 65	0.93 (0.81, 1.08)	1.13 (0.98, 1.30)
Men	1.00 (0.85, 1.18)	1.10 (0.94, 1.29)
Women	0.84 (0.69, 1.03)	1.22 (1.01, 1.46)
Black	0.93 (0.76, 1.14)	1.40 (1.17, 1.68)
Non-Black	0.93 (0.79, 1.10)	1.00 (0.85, 1.17)
Diabetic	0.90 (0.75, 1.08)	1.07 (0.90, 1.28)
Non-Diabetic	0.96 (0.81, 1.14)	1.23 (1.05, 1.44)

Amlodipine Better — Chlorthalidone Better

Lisinopril Better — Chlorthalidone Better

p=0.01 for interaction

Figure 42. Relative risk of stroke according to patient subgroupings in the ALLHAT trial.

ACE inhibitor (-11%) compared to the diuretic. This finding was far more striking in men (-17%) then in women (0%). Of note, blood pressure control was virtually identical between the 2 treatment groups in this study, unlike that of the ALLHAT trial. This may have been due to the lack of black patients in the Australian trial; thus, less of a disparity in BP control would occur in a more homogenous population who lacked as much salt sensitivity and low renin status as was likely to have occurred in ALLHAT.

The final results of these 2 major hypertension trials will be discussed for some time by experts and practicing physicians alike. Clearly, the results of the studies demonstrate that patients must be treated as individuals, that responses to drugs will vary substantially, and that combinations of agents will very often be necessary to avoid the serious complications of hypertension.

Summary

Recent outcome trials provide clear evidence that high-risk patients benefit from blood pressure reduction, intensive antihypertensive drug treatment and "tight" blood pressure control. This applies to the elderly and/or diabetic hypertensive patient and to the patient at high CV risk because of a previous CHD event or stroke. On the basis of the available evidence, it is difficult to discriminate against the "old" drugs, particularly thiazide diuretics, in terms of their proven ability to reduce CV morbidity and mortality. As yet, there is little compelling evidence that the newer drugs, CCBs and ACEIs, which are metabolically "cleaner" and which may have additional non-haemodynamic benefits, can produce superior outcome results.

In current clinical practice there is a clear preference for "established" treatments because they have the greatest volume both of usage and of clinical outcome evidence; thus, low-dose thiazide diuretics (with/without potassium-sparing combinations) and beta-blockers (albeit with some reservations about their overall effectiveness in hypertension) are still widely regarded as first-choice treatments. Increasingly, however, CCBs and ACEIs are considered to be appropriate first-line alternative treatments not only because they are effective and reasonably well tolerated, but also because there is now evidence of benefit from clinical outcome trials, particularly through treatment based upon different dihydropyridine CCBs.

The "alternative" agents, both old and new, may have advantages and this particularly applies to the newer angiotensin II receptor antagonists, which appear to be both effective and particularly well tolerated. This desirable characteristic, allied to the favourable outcomes in the diabetic nephropathy trials and the suggestion of ancillary benefit beyond blood pressure control in the LIFE trial, suggest that these agents may assume much greater importance in the near future.

Finally, with the increasing emphasis on "tight" blood pressure control – particularly in high-risk patients – there is an inevitable requirement for combination treatments. In this respect, the potentially beneficial ancillary properties of particular drug classes may be of secondary importance after the proven benefits of blood pressure reduction *per se*.

Future Developments

Despite the availability of potent and remarkably well tolerated antihypertensive agents, the treatment of hypertension remains an area where there is considerable research activity. This research focuses on: the development of antihypertensive agents with novel mechanisms of action; the identification of genetic factors implicated in the development of atherosclerotic CVD or the response to antihypertensive drug treatment; and the focus on the benefits of combined interventions to reduce the high incidence of CVD.

Novel antihypertensive agents

The development of new antihypertensive agents has tended to focus on seeking new drugs to enhance vasodilator/ natriuretic mechanisms and new drugs to block vaso-constrictor and sodium-retaining mechanisms. Many of the antihypertensive drugs currently undergoing clinical evaluation are focusing on established mechanisms and, in some instances, are refinements of agents whose deficiencies unrelated to their antihypertensive efficacy resulted in termination of the development programme.

Potassium channel openers

Potassium channel openers are believed to hyperpolarize smooth muscle cells by a direct action on the cell membrane. The consequences of this are relaxation of the blood vessels and potassium channel openers therefore act as potent precapillary vasodilators. A number of potassium channel openers have been developed, including nicorandil, pinacidil and cromakalim. Several new compounds are also being evaluated, but to date none appears to represent a useful therapeutic alternative to currently available agents. This may well be a function of the diversity of potassium channels and the fact that most of the available molecules do not appear to offer appropriate or sufficient tissue selectivity.

Renin inhibitors

ACEIs and angiotensin receptor antagonists have demonstrated the antihypertensive benefit of blockade of the renin–angiotensin–aldosterone system (RAAS). Theoretically, these drugs should have an advantage over existing agents in that they target blockade of the RAAS in a highly specific manner, as renin catalyses the first and rate-limiting step of the RAAS cascade by cleaving angiotensinogen to generate the decapeptide angiotensin I. However, the development of appropriate renin inhibitors has proved to be somewhat elusive and clinical experience with them is limited. Most of the development work has focused on the design of peptide analogues of angiotensinogen, many of which contain the amino acid statine found in pepstatin. Substitution at other sites in the molecule determine potency and species selectivity. Although some recently developed compounds exhibit a degree of oral activity, oral bioavailability remains the main problem with these drugs. Thus, until new compounds with improved disposition characteristics have been developed, it is unlikely that renin inhibitors will be shown to have any advantage or even be equivalent to ACEIs and angiotensin receptor antagonists.

Vasopeptidase inhibitors

Inhibitors of neutral endopeptidase (NEP), the major enzymatic pathway for degradation of natriuretic peptides, were developed with the aim of regulating endogenous levels of atrial natriuretic peptide, which is a vasodilatory hormone. When administered alone, NEP inhibitors have a very modest effect on blood pressure, but the demonstration that the combination of an NEP inhibitor and an ACEI produced CV effects greater than those elicited by inhibition of either enzyme alone led to the synthesis of metalloprotease inhibitors which, within a single molecule, inhibit both enzymes.

Omapatrilat is the prototype agent of a class of drugs now known as vasopeptidase inhibitors. Omapatrilat appears to offer similar inhibitory potency of both NEP and ACE. Initial clinical studies showed considerable promise with a potent antihypertensive effect, particularly in African-Americans. However, an incidence of angio-oedema which was higher than that observed with ACEIs in definitive clinical trials has resulted in a decision not to place this agent on the market in the USA. A number of other compounds are under development, including GW660511, MDL100,240, fasidotril and sampatrilat. These compounds differ from the prototype agent with regard to their pharmacokinetic characteristics and their relative inhibitory potencies at ACE and NEP. It thus remains to be seen whether these pharmacological differences will result in the clinical development of a compound which sustains the antihypertensive potency of omapatrilat but avoids the worrying incidence of angio-oedema.

Endothelin antagonists

Endothelin-1 (ET1) is a very potent vasoconstrictor peptide which was discovered in 1988. It acts on ETA receptors in vascular smooth muscle and also stimulates the generation of renin, angiotensin II, aldosterone and adrenaline. It is therefore not surprising that endothelin might be considered to have a role in the pathogenesis of hypertension and, in turn, that selective ET1 antagonists might be useful in the treatment of hypertension.

Bosentan is an orally active, non-peptide, competitive antagonist of both ETA and ETB receptors. Whilst bosentan successfully lowered blood pressure in experimental animal models of hypertension, the antihypertensive efficacy in human hypertension has been less promising, although one study has provided evidence of blood pressure lowering equivalent to that of enalapril. Very recently, a more specific ETA receptor antagonist, darusentan, has been evaluated in a large multi-centre, randomized, double-blind, parallel group dose–response study. The study showed a dose-dependent reduction of both systolic and diastolic blood pressure with darusentan as compared to placebo in patients with moderate hypertension, with no evidence of change in heart rate. Given the recognized detrimental effects of endothelins on heart, kidneys and the vasculature, ETA antagonism seems to offer promise, but as yet this promise is far from being realized.

Novel formulations

Re-formulating existing well-established agents has been shown to have proven benefit in the treatment of hypertension. Thus, for example, the long-acting GITS formulation of nifedipine offers the advantage of a sustained 24-hour duration of antihypertensive effect with a relative absence of reflex tachycardia, which is in stark contrast to the pharmacological characteristics of short-acting nifedipine capsules. However, other potential benefits may be associated with radical new formulations of existing antihypertensive agents. It is often suggested, with good reason, that failure to achieve blood pressure control in individual patients may well be associated with sub-optimal compliance with the treatment regimen. New formulations might therefore offer significant advantage by way of avoiding such problems or alternatively discriminating between the poorly compliant patient and those with "resistant" hypertension. Patch and depot formulations of antihypertensive drugs are currently being developed, and may well prove to be useful additions to the armamentarium of existing agents available for the treatment of hypertension.

Genetics

As discussed earlier, there is little doubt that genetic factors play an important role in the pathogenesis of essential hypertension. The discovery of the genetic determinants of persistent high blood pressure in humans has several potential clinical applications. Advances in genomic science have already allowed the identification of the underlying genetic causes of syndromes implicated in familial hypertension. These include glucocorticoid-remediable aldosteronism, Liddle's syndrome and a syndrome of apparent mineralocorticoid excess. Linkage analysis in families segregating for rare Mendelian forms of hypertension, candidate gene approaches and genome-wide scanning are three strategies which have been used in the last decade to investigate the causes of inherited hypertension. The major advance must lie in the anticipated results of pharmacogenomics, which it is hoped will identify individuals who would benefit from specific therapies. To date, the use of therapeutic approaches founded upon phenotypic expression such as plasma renin activity have largely been unrewarding. However, a recent double-blind, placebo-controlled crossover comparison of five classes of antihypertensive drugs demonstrated that patients varied reproducibly in their response to initial therapy and that switching among drugs can predictably increase the efficacy of monotherapy.

It is anticipated that, ultimately, genomic research will lead to the detection of major susceptibility and severity genes for hypertension and its vascular complications, providing diagnostic markers for individuals at highest risk. This could lead to the development of novel antihypertensive drugs and may allow intervention before irreversible structural changes have occurred.

Multiple risk factors

As was acknowledged in the introduction of this book, the treatment of hypertension rarely occurs in isolation and in general should be considered in the context of control of overall CV risk. Whilst the interaction of these risk factors has been documented and is widely appreciated, the most appropriate strategies for the combined treatment are less well understood. For example, it is only very recently that the results of the MRC/BHF Heart Protection Study have demonstrated the value of adding the HMG CoA reductase inhibitor, simvastatin, to existing treatment in patients at high risk of CV complications, irrespective of their initial cholesterol concentrations (Figures 43 and 44).[58] Thus, further insight needs to be gained into which patients stand to benefit from targeting overall CV risk and what treatment thresholds are appropriate for these combined risks

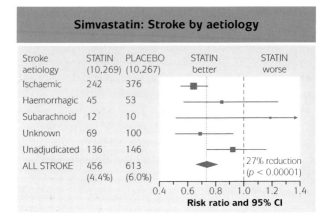

Figure 43. Results of the HPS trial: the benefits by way of stroke reduction associated with simvastatin treatment. Data from reference 56.

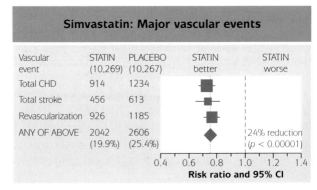

Figure 44. Results of the HPS trial: the reduction in major vascular events associated with simvastatin treatment. Data from reference 56.

Frequently Asked Questions

I have been diagnosed as having high blood pressure. Why should I bother with treatment?
Having high blood pressure increases your risk of heart attack, stroke and other conditions. Treatment has been shown to considerably reduce this risk.

What are the symptoms of high blood pressure?
Usually none, unless BP is very high for a protracted period. Contrary to popular belief, the normal day-to-day fluctuations in BP are asymptomatic. Correspondingly, headache is seldom a feature of the usual type of mild to moderate hypertension.

What causes high blood pressure?
In most cases (95%) there is no clearly identifiable cause, although genetic factors (family history) and environmental factors (e.g. obesity, excessive alcohol intake) are contributory.

How common is hypertension?
It affects about 15–20% of the general population but it increases in prevalence with increasing age.

If I have high blood pressure will I have to take drugs to lower it?
Yes – in most cases. In some cases, however, effective lifestyle modification (weight reduction and increased physical activity, for example) can obviate the need for drug treatment, or reduce the number of drugs required.

Will having hypertension affect my ability to get life insurance?
Not if the BP is well controlled. In the USA, it might affect rate/premiums.

My father died of a heart attack when he was 51. Will treating my high blood pressure stop me having a heart attack?

Medical treatment for any condition does not guarantee a "cure", but the chances of a heart attack are markedly reduced and, if it does occur, it is likely to be delayed to a significantly older age.

Will having high blood pressure mean that I will not be able to keep working?

For most occupations, controlled hypertension will not prevent you from working. This particularly applies if you fly, work as a diver or drive vehicles over 3.5 tonnes (or a minibus with more than eight seats).

I have high blood pressure. Can I donate blood?

No…because drug treatments will be present in your blood. In the USA, however, hypertensives can donate blood.

If I have high blood pressure will my children suffer from it?

No, not necessarily, although their chances will be higher because of the family history. Even if there is a family history, the chances of having high blood pressure are reduced by a healthy lifestyle.

If I am diagnosed as having high blood pressure, how often should I see my doctor?

This is an individual issue, but once the condition is assessed and effectively treated the visits can typically be 6- or 12-monthly.

What should I do if I forget to take my tablets for 1 or 2 days?

Simply restart the regular dosage (do not try to "catch up" by taking extra doses) and resolve never again to omit the medicines!

If my blood pressure is controlled for a long time, will I be able to stop taking my antihypertensive drugs?

As a general rule, no. Only if there has been substantial lifestyle improvement through, for example, significant weight loss and increased physical activity is this likely.

I have been smoking 20 cigarettes a day for over 25 years. Is there any benefit in stopping now or is it too late?

It is never too late to stop smoking. Even for people who have had a heart attack, the chances of a further heart problem are halved if smoking is stopped.

Do nicotine patches or chewing gum increase blood pressure?

Not to any significant extent, although it is important to continue with your regular BP treatment.

Will having high blood pressure affect my sex life?

Hypertension itself will not affect sexual activity. Sexual activity does raise your blood pressure, but only briefly, and if your blood pressure has been controlled, this does not confer any risk.

Some of the drug treatments can occasionally cause problems, particularly for men, but adjustment of the drug treatment will usually resolve this. Don't some blood pressure-lowering drugs cause impotence?

Yes…but the likeliest culprits can be avoided or replaced with alternatives.

I have heard that alcohol is good for heart disease. Will it help my blood pressure?

Alcohol in moderation appears to be beneficial. Excessive consumption may itself be a cause of hypertension.

I have high blood pressure. Do I have to give up playing sports?

No…but probably best to wait until the treatment is stabilized if high intensity isometric sports (e.g. weightlifting) are being considered.

Will the contraceptive pill affect my blood pressure?

Some contraceptive pills can cause a small rise in blood pressure. Therefore, if you have high blood pressure your doctor will not recommend the "combined pill". In some instances you may be asked to consider other forms of contraception.

Does stress cause high blood pressure?

Although stressful situations may cause your blood pressure to rise, this is only for a short time, and once stress is relieved blood pressure returns to normal. This is the normal pattern in everyone and is unlikely to be a cause of sustained high blood pressure.

References

1. Burt VL, Whelton P, Rocceila E *et al*. Prevalence of hypertension in the US adult population: results from the third National Health and Nutrition Examination Survey, 1988–1991. *Hypertension* 1995; **25**: 305–313.

2. Mancia G, Sega R, Milesi C, Cesana G, Zanchetti A. Blood-pressure control in the hypertensive population. *Lancet* 1997; **349**: 454–457.

3. Primatesta P, Brookes M, Poulter NR. Improved Hypertension Management Control. Results from the Health Survey for England 1998. *Hypertension* 2001; **38**: 827–832.

4. Isles CG, Walker LM, Beevers DG *et al*. Mortality in patients of the Glasgow Blood Pressure Clinic. *J Hypertens* 1986; **4**: 141–156.

5. McMahon S, Peto R, Cutler J *et al*. Blood pressure, stroke and CHD, Part 1. Prolonged differences in blood pressure: prospective observational studies collected for the regression dilution bias. *Lancet* 1990; **335**: 765–774.

6. Joint National Committee on Prevention, Detection, Evaluation and Treatment of High Blood Pressure. The sixth report of the Joint National Committee on Prevention, Detection, Evaluation and Treatment of High Blood Pressure. *Arch Intern Med* 1997; **157**: 2413–2446.

7. Guidelines Subcommittee. 1999 World Health Organisation–International Society of Hypertension guidelines for the management of hypertension. *J Hypertens* 1999; **17**: 151–183.

8. Glen SK, Elliott HL, Curzio JL, Lees KR, Reid JL. White coat hypertension as a cause of cardiovascular dysfunction. *Lancet* 1996; **348**: 654–657.

9. Bidlingmeyer I, Burnier M, Bidlingmeyer M, Waeber B, Brunner HR. Isolated office hypertension: a prehypertensive state? *J Hypertens* 1996; **14**: 327–332.

10. Kannel WB, Gordon T, Schwartz MJ. Systolic versus diastolic blood pressure and risk of coronary heart disease: The Framingham Study. *Am J Cardiol* 1971; **27**: 335–345.

11. Verdecchia P, Schillaci G, Borgioni C, Ciucci A, Pede S, Porcellati C. Ambulatory pulse pressure. A potent predictor of total cardiovascular risk in hypertension. *Hypertension* 1998; **32**: 983–988.

12. Blacher J, Staessen JA, Girerd X *et al*. Pulse pressure not mean pressure determines cardiovascular risk in older hypertensive patients. *Arch Intern Med* 2000; **160**: 1085–1089.

13. Klag MJ, Whelton PK, Randall BL, Neaton JD, Brancati FL, Stamler J. End-stage renal disease in African-American and white men. 16-year MRFIT findings. *JAMA* 1997; **277**: 1293–1298.

14. Cruikshank JK, Beevers DG, Osbourne VL *et al*. Heart attack, stroke, diabetes and hypertension in West Indians, Asians and Whites in Birmingham, England. *Br Med J* 1980; **281**: 1108.

15. Reaven GM. Role of insulin resistance in human disease: Banting Lecture. *Diabetes* 1988; **37**: 1595–1607.

16. Shore AC, Markandu ND, MacGregor GA. A randomized crossover study to compare the blood pressure response to sodium loading with and without chloride in patients with essential hypertension. *J Hypertens*. 1998; **6**: 613–617.

17. Vriz O, Piccolo D, Cozzutti E *et al*. on behalf of the HARVEST Study Group. The effects of alcohol consumption on ambulatory blood pressure and target organs in subjects with borderline to mild hypertension. *Am J Hypertens* 1998; **11**: 230–234.

18. Cappuccio FP, MacGregor GA. Does potassium supplementation lower blood pressure? A meta-analysis of published trials. *J Hypertens* 1991; **9**: 465–473.

19. Cappuccio FP, Siani A, Strazullo P. Oral calcium supplementation and blood pressure: an overview of randomised controlled trials. *J Hypertens* 1989; **7**: 941–946.

20. Pripp U, Hall G, Csemiczky G *et al*. A randomised trial on effects of hormone therapy on ambulatory blood pressure and lipoprotein levels in women with coronary artery disease. *J Hypertens* 1999; **17**: 1379–1386.

21. Harvey PJ, Wing LM, Savage J, Molloy D. The effects of different types and doses of oestrogen replacement therapy on clinic and ambulatory blood pressure and the renin–angiotensin system in normotensive and postmenopausal women. *J Hypertens* 1999; **17**: 405–414.

22. Wolf PA, D'Agostino RB, Belanger AJ, Kannel WB. Probability of stroke: A risk profile from the Framingham Study. *Stroke* 1991; **22**: 312–318.

23. Actuarial Society of America and the Association of Life Insurance Medical Directors. *Supplement to blood pressure study*. New York: Actuarial Society of America and the Association of Life Insurance Medical Directors, 1941.

24. Wilson PWF, Kannel WB. Hypertension, other risk factors and risk of cardiovascular disease. In: Laragh JH, Brenner BM, editors. *Hypertension: Pathophysiology, Diagnosis and Management*, 2nd Edition. New York: Raven Press, New York , 1995; pp. 99–114.

25. Vasan RS, Larson MG, Leip EP, Kannel WB, Levy D. Assessment of progression to hypertension in non-hypertensive participants in the Framingham Heart Study: a cohort study. *Lancet* 2001; **358**: 1682–1686.

26. Anderson KM, Odell PM, Wilson PWF, Kannel WB, Cardiovascular disease risk profiles. *Am Heart J* 1990; **121**: 293–829.

27. Lip GYH, Beevers M, Beevers DG. Complications and survival of 315 patients with malignant-phase hypertension. *J Hypertens* 1995; **13**: 915–924.

28. Robertson JIS, Ball SG. Treating hypertension. In: *Hypertension for the Clinician*. London: WB Saunders Co Ltd, 1994; pp. 101–111.

29. Collins R, McMahon S. Blood pressure, antihypertensive drug treatment and the risks of stroke and coronary heart disease. *Br Med Bull* 1994; **50**: 272–298.

30. Ramsay LE, Williams B, Johnston GD *et al*. British Hypertension Society guidelines for hypertension management 1999: summary. *BMJ* 1999; **319**: 630–635.

31. Perloff D, Sokolow M, Cowan R. The prognostic value of ambulatory blood pressures. *JAMA* 1983; **249**: 2792–2798.

32. White WB, Dey HM, Schulman P. Assessment of the daily blood pressure load as a determinant of cardiac function in patients with mild–moderate hypertension. *Am Heart J* 1989; **118**: 782–795.

33. SHEP Co-operative Research Group. Prevention of stroke by antihypertensive drug treatment in older persons with isolated systolic hypertension: Final results of the Systolic Hypertension in the Elderly Program (SHEP). *JAMA* 1991; **265**: 3255–3264.

34. Staessen JA, Gasowski J, Wang JG *et al*. Risks of untreated systolic hypertension in the elderly: meta-analysis of outcome trials. *Lancet* 2000; **355**: 865–872.

35. Hansson L, Zanchetti A, Carruthers SG *et al*. for the HOT study group. Effects of intensive blood pressure lowering and low-dose aspirin in patients with hypertension: principal results to the Hypertension Optimal Study (HOT) randomised trial. *Lancet* 1998; **351**: 1755–1762.

36. The Heart Outcomes Prevention Evaluation Study Investigators. Effects of an angiotensin-converting-enzyme inhibitor, ramipril, on cardiovascular events in high-risk patients. *New Engl J Med* 2000; **342**: 145–153.

37. PROGRESS Collaborative group. Randomised trial of a perindopril-based blood-pressure-lowering regimen among 6105 individuals with previous stroke or transient ischaemic attack. *Lancet* 2001; **358**: 1033–1041.

38. Gueyffier E, Bulpitt C, Boisel JP *et al.* for the INDANA Group. Antihypertensive drugs in very old people: a sub-group meta-analysis of randomised controlled trials. *Lancet* 1999; **353**: 793–796.

39. Appel LJ, Moore TJ, Obarzanek E *et al.* for the DASH Collaborative Research Group. A clinical trial of the effects of dietary patterns on blood pressure. *New Engl J Med* 1997; **336**: 1117–1124.

40. Whelton PK, Appel LJ, Espeland MA *et al.* for the TONE Collaborative Research Group. Sodium reduction and weight loss in the treatment of hypertension in older persons. A randomized controlled trial of nonpharmacologic interventions in the elderly (TONE). *JAMA* 1998; **279**: 839–846.

41. White WB, Kent J, Taylor A, Verburg KM, Lefkowith JB, Whelton A. Effects of celecoxib on ambulatory blood pressure in hypertensive patients on ACE inhibitors. *Hypertension* 2002; **39**(4): 929–934.

42. Conlin PR, Gerth WC, Fox J *et al.* Four-year persistence patterns among patients initiating therapy with the angiotensin II receptor antagonist losartan versus other antihypertensive drug classes. Clin Ther 2001; 23(12): 1999–2010.

43. ALLHAT Collaborative Research Group. Major cardiovascular events in hypertensive patients randomized to doxazosin vs chlorthalidone: the antihypertensive and lipid-lowering treatment to prevent heart attack trial (ALLHAT). *JAMA* 2000; **283**: 1967–1975.

44. Staessen JA, Fagard R, Thijs L *et al.* A randomised doubleblind comparison of placebo and active treatment for older patients with isolated systolic hypertension. *Lancet* 1997; **350**: 757–64.

45. UK Prospective Diabetes Study Group. Tight blood pressure control and risk of macrovascular and microvascular complications in type II diabetes: UKPDS 38. *BMJ* 1998; **317**: 703–713.

46. Hansson L, Lindholm LH, Niskanen L *et al.* for the Captopril Prevention Project (CAPPP) study group. Effect of angiotensin-converting enzyme inhibition compared with conventional therapy on cardio-

vascular morbidity and mortality in hypertension: the Captopril Prevention Project (CAPP) randomised trial. *Lancet* 1999; **353**: 611–616.

47. Hansson L, Lindholm LH, Ekbom R *et al*. Randomised trial of old and new antihypertensive drugs in elderly patients: cardiovascular mortality and morbidity the Swedish Trial in Old Patients with Hypertension-2 Study. *Lancet* 1999; **354**: 1751–1756.

48. Brown MJ, Palmer CR, Castaigne A *et al*. Morbidity and mortality in patients randomised to double-blind treatment with a long-acting calcium-channel blocker or diuretic in the International Nifedipine GITS study: intervention as a goal in hypertension treatment (INSIGHT). *Lancet* 2000; **356**: 366–372.

49. Hansson L, Hedner T, Lund–Johansen P, Kjeldsen SE, Lindholm LH, Syvertsen JO for the NORDIL Study Group. Randomized trial of effects of calcium antagonists compared with diuretics and β-blockers on cardio-vascular morbidity and mortality in hypertension: the Nordic Diltiazem (NORDIL) study for the NORDIL Study Group. *Lancet* 2000; **356**: 339–365.

50. Blood Pressure Lowering Treatment Trialists' Collaboration. Effects of ACE inhibitors, calcium antagonists, and other blood-pressure-lowering drugs: results of prospectively designed overviews of randomized trials. *Lancet* 2000; **356**: 1955–1964.

51. Pahor M, Psaty BM, Alderman MH *et al*. Health outcomes associated with calcium antagonists compared with other first-line antihypertensive therapies: a meta-analysis of randomised controlled trials. *Lancet* 2000; **356**: 1949–1954.

52. Brenner BM, Cooper ME, de Zeeuw D *et al*. Effects of losartan on renal and cardiovascular outcomes in patients with type II diabetes and nephropathy. *N Engl J Med* 2001; **345**: 861–9.

53. Lewis EJ, Hunsicker LG, Clarke WR *et al*. Renoprotective effect of the angiotensin-receptor antagonist irbesartan in patients with nephropathy due to type II diabetes. *New Engl J Med* 2001; **345**: 851–860.

54. Parving H, Lehnert H, Brochner–Mortensen J, Gomis R, Andersen S, Asner P. The effect of irbesartan on the development of diabetic nephropathy on patients with type II diabetes. *New Engl J Me*d 2001; **345**: 870–878.

55. Dahlof B, Devereux RB, Kjeldsen SE *et al*. Cardiovascular morbidity and mortality in the Losartan Intervention For Endpoint reduction in hypertension study (LIFE): a randomized trial against atenolol. *Lancet* 2002; **359**: 995–1003,

56. The ALLHAT Officers and Coordinators for the ALLHAT Collaborative Research Group. Major outcomes in high-risk hypertensive patients randomised to angiotensin-converting enzyme inhibitor or CCB vs. diuretic: the Antihypertensive and Lipid Lowering Treatment to Prevent Heart Attack Trial (ALLHAT). *JAMA* 2002; **288**: 2981-2997.

57. Wing LMH, Reid CM, Ryan P, Beilin LJ, Brown MA, Jennings GLR, et al. A comparison of outcomes with angiotensin-converting enzyme inhibitors and diuretics for hypertension in the elderly. *New Engl J Med* 2003; **348**: 583-592.

58. Heart Protection Study Collaborative Group. MRC/BHF Heart Protection Study of cholesterol lowering with simvastatin in 20536 high-risk individuals: a randomized placebo-controlled trial. *Lancet* 2002; **360**: 7–22.

Appendix 1 – Drugs

Drug	Trade name	Preparation	Strength	Doses used in hypertension (adult)	Comments	Side-effects
Thiazide diuretics						
Bendroflumethiazide (bendrofluazide)	Neo-NaClex	Tablet	2.5, 5 mg	2.5 mg mane	Drug of choice for elderly patients; contraindicated in patients with gout; caution in hepatic and renal impairment, pregnancy and breast feeding	Postural hypotension, mild gastrointestinal effects, impotence, hypokalaemia, hypomagnesaemia, hyponatraemia, hypocalcaemia, hypochloraemic alkalosis, hyperuricaemia, gout, hyperglycaemia, altered plasma lipid concentrations
Bendroflumethiazide + potassium	Centyl K	Tablet	2.5 mg + 8.4 mmol	1 tablet mane	Combination of thiazide and potassium-sparing diuretics preferable; swallow whole with plenty of water	
	Neo-NaClex-K	Tablet	2.5 mg + 7.7 mmol	1 tablet mane		
Chlortalidone (chlorthalidone)	Hygroton	Tablet	50 mg	25 mg mane increasing to 50 mg prn	Drug of choice for elderly patients; contraindicated in patients with gout; caution in hepatic and renal impairment, pregnancy and breast feeding	Postural hypotension, mild gastrointestinal effects, impotence, hypokalaemia, hypomagnesaemia, hyponatraemia, hypocalcaemia, hypochloraemic alkalosis, hyperuricaemia, gout, hyperglycaemia, altered plasma lipid concentrations

Drug	Trade name	Preparation	Strength	Doses used in hypertension (adult)	Comments	Side-effects
Thiazide diuretics						
Cyclopen-thiazide	Navidrex	Capsule	500 mcg	250 mcg mane increasing to 500 mcg prn	Drug of choice for elderly patients; contraindicated in patients with gout; use with other drugs if hypertension is not controlled with low dose	Postural hypotension, mild gastrointestinal effects, impotence, hypokalaemia, hypomagnesaemia, hyponatraemia, hypocalcaemia, hypochloraemic alkalosis, hyperuricaemia, gout, hyperglycaemia, altered plasma lipid concentrations
Hydrochloro-thiazide	HydroSaluric	Tablet	25, 50 mg	25 mg mane increasing to 50 mg prn	Drug of choice for elderly patients; contraindicated in patients with gout; caution in hepatic and renal impairment, pregnancy and breast feeding	Postural hypotension, mild gastrointestinal effects, impotence, hypokalaemia, hypomagnesaemia, hyponatraemia, hypocalcaemia, hypochloraemic alkalosis, hyperuricaemia, gout, hyperglycaemia, altered plasma lipid concentrations
Indapamide	Natrilix	Tablet	2.5 mg	2.5 mg mane	Drug of choice for elderly patients; contraindicated in patients with gout; caution in hepatic and renal impairment, pregnancy and breast feeding	Hypokalaemia, headache, dizziness, fatigue, muscle cramps, nausea, anorexia, diarrhoea, constipation, rashes
	Natrilix SR	M/R tablet	1.5 mg (1.25 mg for Lozol)	1.5 mg mane		
Metolazone	Metenix 5	Tablet	5 mg	5 mg mane; maintenance 5 mg on alternate days	Drug of choice for elderly patients; contraindicated in patients with gout; caution in hepatic and renal impairment, pregnancy and breast feeding	Postural hypotension, mild gastrointestinal effects, impotence, hypokalaemia, hypomagnesaemia, hyponatraemia, hypocalcaemia, hypochloraemic alkalosis, hyperuricaemia, gout, hyperglycaemia, altered plasma lipid concentrations

Drug	Trade name	Preparation	Strength	Doses used in hypertension (adult)	Comments	Side-effects
Thiazide diuretics						
Polythiazide	Nephril	Tablet	1 mg	500 mcg mane	Drug of choice for elderly patients; contraindicated in patients with gout; caution in hepatic and renal impairment, pregnancy and breast feeding	Postural hypotension, mild gastrointestinal effects, impotence, hypokalaemia, hypomagnesaemia, hyponatraemia, hypocalcaemia, hypochloraemic alkalosis, hyperuricaemia, gout, hyperglycaemia, altered plasma lipid concentrations
Xipamide	Diurexan	Tablet	20 mg	20 mg mane	Drug of choice for elderly patients; contraindicated in patients with gout; caution in hepatic and renal impairment, pregnancy and breast feeding	Gastrointestinal effects, mild dizziness, hypokalaemia and other electrolyte disturbances
Loop diuretics						
Furosemide (frusemide)	Lasix	Tablet / Liquid	20, 40, 80 mg / 1 mg/ml	20–40 mg mane	Used to lower blood pressure in patients with chronic renal failure who have not responded to thiazide diuretics; caution in pregnancy and breast feeding	Hyponatraemia, hypokalaemia, hypomagnesaemia, hypochloraemic alkalosis, increased calcium excretion
Bumetanide	Burinex	Tablet / Liquid	1, 5 mg / 1 mg/5 ml	1 mg mane	Used to lower blood pressure in patients with chronic renal failure who have not responded to thiazide diuretics; caution in pregnancy and breast feeding	Hyponatraemia, hypokalaemia, hypomagnesaemia, hypochloraemic alkalosis, increased calcium excretion, myalgia

Drug	Trade name	Preparation	Strength	Doses used in hypertension (adult)	Comments	Side-effects
Loop diuretics						
Torasemide	Torem	Tablet	2.5, 5, 10 mg	2.5 mg mane increasing to 5 mg prn	Used to lower blood pressure in patients with chronic renal failure who have not responded to thiazide diuretics; caution in pregnancy and breast feeding	Hyponatraemia, hypokalaemia, hypomagnesaemia, hypochloraemic alkalosis, increased calcium excretion, dry mouth
Potassium-sparing diuretics (with other diuretics)						
Amiloride	Generic	Tablet	5 mg	5–10 mg mane	Used in combination with thiazide diuretics to treat hypertension; contraindicated in renal failure; caution in diabetes mellitus, pregnancy and breast feeding	Gastrointestinal effects, dry mouth, rashes, confusion, postural hypotension, hyperkalaemia, hyponatraemia
Amiloride + cyclopenthiazide	Navispare	Tablet	2.5 mg + 250 mcg	1–2 tablets mane		See also cyclopenthiazide
Amiloride + hydrochlorothiazide (co-amilozide)	Moduret 25	Tablet	2.5 + 25 mg	2.5 + 25–5 + 50 mg mane (max 5 + 50 mane)		See also hydrochlorothiazide
	Moduretic		5 + 50 mg			

Drug	Trade name	Preparation	Strength	Doses used in hypertension (adult)	Comments	Side-effects
Potassium-sparing diuretics (with other diuretics)						
Triamterene	Dytac	Capsule	50 mg	150–250 mg daily (less with thiazide diuretics), maintenance 150–250 mg on alternate days	Used in combination with thiazide diuretics to treat hypertension; contraindicated in renal failure; caution in diabetes mellitus, pregnancy and breast feeding; take with or after food	Gastrointestinal effects, dry mouth, rashes, hyperkalaemia, hyponatraemia
Triamterene + hydrochlorothiazide (co-triamterzide)	Dyazide	Tablet	37.5 + 25 mg	1 tablet mane (max 4 tablets/day);		See also hydrochlorothiazide
Triamterene + chlortalidone	Kalspare	Tablet	50 + 50 mg	1–2 tablets mane		See also chlortalidone
Beta-adrenoceptor blocking drugs						
Acebutolol	Sectral	Capsule / Tablet	400 mg/day increasing to 400 mg 2 times/day prn	400 mg/day increasing to 400 mg 2 times/day prn	Contraindicated in asthma, chronic obstructive pulmonary disease and heart block; caution in renal and hepatic impairment, pregnancy and breast feeding	Bradycardia (less likely), heart failure, conduction disorders, bronchospasm, peripheral vasoconstriction (less likely), gastrointestinal effects, fatigue, sleep disturbance
Acebutolol + hydrochlorothiazide	Secadrex	Tablet	1–2 tablets mane	1–2 tablets mane		See also hydrochlorothiazide

Beta-adrenoceptor blocking drugs

Drug	Trade name	Preparation	Strength	Doses used in hypertension (adult)	Comments	Side-effects
Atenolol	Tenormin 25	Tablet	25 mg	25–200 mg/day	Contraindicated in asthma, chronic obstructive pulmonary disease and heart block; accumulates in renal impairment (reduce dose); caution in hepatic impairment, pregnancy and breast feeding	Bradycardia, heart failure, conduction disorders, bronchospasm, peripheral vasoconstriction, gastrointestinal effects, fatigue, sleep disturbance (less likely)
	Tenormin LS	Tablet	50 mg			
	Tenormin	Tablet	100 mg			
Atenolol + bendroflu-methazide	Tenben	Capsule	25 + 1.25 mg	25 + 1.25 mane		See also bendroflumethazide
Atenolol + chlortalidone (co-tenidone)	Tenoret 50	Tablet	50 + 12.5 mg	50 + 12.5–100 + 25 mane		See also chlortalidone
	Tenoretic	Tablet	100 + 25 mg			
Atenolol + amiloride + hydrochloro-thiazide	Kalten	Capsule	50 + 2.5 + 25 mg	1 capsule mane	Only indicated when calcium channel blocker or beta-blocker alone is inadequate; swallow whole	See also amiloride and hydrochlorothiazide
	Beta-Adalat	M/R capsule	50 + 20 mg	1–2 capsules/day (elderly 1 capsule/day)		
Atenolol + nifedipine	Tenif	M/R capsule	50 + 20 mg	1–2 capsules/day (elderly 1 capsule/day)		See also nifedipine

Drug	Trade name	Preparation	Strength	Doses used in hypertension (adult)	Comments	Side-effects
Beta-adrenoceptor blocking drugs						
Betaxolol	Kerlone	Tablet	20 mg	20–40 mg/day (elderly 10 mg/day)	Contraindicated in asthma, chronic obstructive pulmonary disease and heart block; relatively cardioselective; accumulates in renal impairment (reduce dose); caution in hepatic impairment, pregnancy and breast feeding	Bradycardia, heart failure, conduction disorders, bronchospasm, peripheral vasoconstriction, gastrointestinal effects, fatigue, sleep disturbance
Bisoprolol	Cardicor	Tablet	2.5, 5 mg	5–10 mg/day (max 20 mg/day)	Contraindicated in asthma, chronic obstructive pulmonary disease and heart block; relatively cardioselective; accumulates in hepatic and renal impairment (reduce dose); caution in pregnancy and breast feeding	radycardia, heart failure, conduction disorders, bronchospasm, peripheral vasoconstriction, gastrointestinal effects, fatigue, sleep disturbance
	Emcor	Tablet	5, 10 mg			
	Monocor	Tablet	5, 10 mg			
Bisoprolol + hydrochlorothiazide	Monozide 10	Tablet	10 + 0.25 mg (2.5 or 5 + 6.25 mg for Ziac)	1 tablet/day		BSee also hydrochlorothiazide

Beta-adrenoceptor blocking drugs

Drug	Trade name	Preparation	Strength	Doses used in hypertension (adult)	Comments	Side-effects
Carvedilol	Eucardic	Tablet	3.125, 6.25, 12.5, 25 mg	12.5–25 mg/day (elderly 12.5 mg/day) (max 50 mg/day)	Contraindicated in asthma, chronic obstructive pulmonary disease, heart block and hepatic impairment; caution in renal impairment, pregnancy and breast feeding	Postural hypotension, dizziness, headache, fatigue, gastrointestinal effects, bradycardia
Celiprolol	Celectol	Tablet	200, 400 mg	200 mg mane increasing to 400 mg pm	Contraindicated in asthma, chronic obstructive pulmonary disease and heart block; accumulates in renal impairment (reduce dose); caution in hepatic impairment, pregnancy and breast feeding; take before food	Headache, dizziness, fatigue, nausea, somnolence
Labetolol	Trandate	Tablet	100, 200, 400 mg	100–200 mg 2 times/day (elderly 50 mg 2 times/day initially) (max 2.4 g/day)	Contraindicated in asthma, chronic obstructive pulmonary disease, heart block and hepatic impairment; caution in renal impairment, pregnancy and breast feeding; take with or after food	Postural hypotension, tiredness, weakness, headache, rashes, scalp tingling, difficulty in micturition, epigastric pain, nausea, vomiting, liver damage
Metoprolol	Betaloc	Tablet	50, 100 mg	100 mg/day; maintenance 100–200 mg/day	Contraindicated in asthma, chronic obstructive pulmonary disease, heart block; accumulates in hepatic impairment (reduce dose); caution in hepatic impairment, pregnancy and breast feeding; M/R formulations should be swallowed whole	Bradycardia, heart failure, conduction disorders, bronchospasm, peripheral vasoconstriction, gastrointestinal effects, fatigue, sleep disturbance
	Betaloc-SA	M/R tablet	200 mg			
	Lopressor	Tablet	50, 100 mg			

Beta-adrenoceptor blocking drugs

Drug	Trade name	Preparation	Strength	Doses used in hypertension (adult)	Comments	Side-effects
Metoprolol cont...	Lopressor SR	M/R tablet	25, 50, 100, 200 mg			
Metoprolol + hydrochloro-thiazide	Co-Betaloc	Tablet	50/100 + 12.5 mg	1–3 tablets/day		
	Co-Betaloc SA	M/R tablet	200 + 25 mg	1 tablet/day		See also hydrochlorothiazide
Nadolol	Corgard	Tablet	40, 80 mg	80 mg/day (max 240 mg/day)	Contraindicated in asthma, chronic obstructive pulmonary disease and heart block; caution in renal and hepatic impairment, pregnancy and breast feeding	Bradycardia, heart failure, conduction disorders, bronchospasm, peripheral vasoconstriction, gastrointestinal effects, fatigue, sleep disturbance (less likely)
Nadolol + bendroflu-methazide	Corgaretic	M/R tablet	40 + 5, 80 + 5 mg	1–2 tablets/day		See also bendroflumethazide

Drug	Trade name	Preparation	Strength	Doses used in hypertension (adult)	Comments	Side-effects
Beta-adrenoceptor blocking drugs						
Nebivolol	Nebilet	Tablet	5 mg	5 mg/day (2.5 mg/day initially elderly)	Contraindicated in asthma, chronic obstructive pulmonary disease, heart block and hepatic impairment; accumulates in renal impairment (reduce dose); caution in pregnancy and breast feeding	Bradycardia, heart failure, conduction disorders, bronchospasm, peripheral vasoconstriction, gastrointestinal effects, fatigue, sleep disturbance, oedema, headache, depression, visual disturbances, impotence
Oxprenolol	Trasicor	Tablet	20, 40, 80 mg	80–160 mg/day in 2–3 divided doses (max 320 mg)	Contraindicated in asthma, chronic obstructive pulmonary disease and heart block; caution in renal and hepatic impairment, pregnancy and breast feeding; M/R formulation should be swallowed whole	Bradycardia (less likely), heart failure, conduction disorders, bronchospasm, peripheral vasoconstriction (less likely), gastrointestinal effects, fatigue, sleep disturbance
	Slow-Trasicor	M/R tablet	160 mg	160 mg/day (max 320 mg/day)		
Oxprenolol + cyclopenthiazide (co-prenozide)	Trasidrex	Tablet	160 mg + 250 mcg	1 tablet mane (max 2 tablets mane)		See also cyclopenthiazide
Pindolol	Visken	Tablet	5, 15 mg	5 mg 2–3 times/day increasing to 15–30 mg/day (max 45 mg/day)	Contraindicated in asthma, chronic obstructive pulmonary disease, heart block; accumulates in renal impairment (reduce dose); caution in hepatic impairment, pregnancy and breast feeding	Bradycardia, heart failure, conduction disorders, bronchospasm, peripheral vasoconstriction, gastrointestinal effects, fatigue, sleep disturbance
Pindolol + clopamide	Viskaldix	Tablet	10 + 5 mg	1–2 mane (max 3 mane)		

Drug	Trade name	Preparation	Strength	Doses used in hypertension (adult)	Comments	Side-effects
Beta-adrenoceptor blocking drugs						
Propranolol	Inderal	Tablet	10, 40, 80 mg	80 mg 2 times/day; maintenance 160–320 mg/day	Contraindicated in asthma, chronic obstructive pulmonary disease and heart block; caution in renal and hepatic impairment, pregnancy and breast feeding; M/R formulations should be swallowed whole	Bradycardia, heart failure, conduction disorders, bronchospasm, peripheral vasoconstriction, gastrointestinal effects, fatigue, sleep disturbance
	Half-Inderal LA	M/R capsule	80 mg	80–160 mg/day		
	Inderal LA	M/R capsule	80, 160 mg	160–320 mg/day		
Propranolol + bendroflumethazide	Inderetic	Capsule	80 + 2.5 mg	1 capsule 2 times/day		See also bendroflumethazide
	Inderex	M/R capsule	160 + 5 mg	1 capsule/day		
Timolol	Betim	Tablet	5, 10 mg	10 mg/day (max 60 mg/day in divided doses if above 20 mg)	Contraindicated in asthma, chronic obstructive pulmonary disease and heart block; caution in renal and hepatic impairment, pregnancy and breast feeding	Bradycardia, heart failure, conduction disorders, bronchospasm, peripheral vasoconstriction, gastrointestinal effects, fatigue, sleep disturbance

Drug	Trade name	Preparation	Strength	Doses used in hypertension (adult)	Comments	Side-effects
Beta-adrenoceptor blocking drugs						
Timolol + amiloride + hydrochlorothiazide	Moducren	Tablet	10 + 2.5 + 25 mg	1–2 tablets mane		See also amiloride and hydrochlorothiazide
Timolol + bendroflumethazide	Prestim	Tablet	10 + 2.5 mg	1–2 tablets mane (max 4 tablets mane)		See also bendrofluethazide
Vasodilator antihypertensive drugs						
Hydralazine	Apresoline	Tablet	25, 50 mg	25 mg 2 times/day increasing to 50 mg 2 times/day prn	Contraindicated in idiopathic systemic lupus erythematosus, severe tachycardia, high output heart failure, myocardial insufficiency due to mechanical obstruction, cor pulmonale, dissecting aortic aneurysm, porphyria; caution in hepatic and renal impairment, pregnancy and breast feeding	Tachycardia, palpitations, flushing, fluid retention, gastrointestinal effects
Minoxidil	Loniten	Tablet	2.5, 5 mg	5 mg/day (2.5 mg/day elderly) (max 50 mg/day)	Contraindicated in phaeochromocytoma; caution in pregnancy	Sodium and water retention, weight gain, peripheral oedema, tachycardia, hypertrichosis

Drug	Trade name	Preparation	Strength	Doses used in hypertension (adult)	Comments	Side-effects
Centrally acting antihypertensive drugs						
Clonidine	Catapres	Tablet	100, 200, 300 mcg	50–100 mcg 3 times/day (max 1.2 mg/day)	Withdraw gradually to avoid hypertensive crisis	Dry mouth, sedation, depression, fluid retention, bradycardia, occlusive peripheral vascular disease, headache, dizziness, euphoria, rash, nausea, constipation
Methyldopa	Aldomet	Tablet	125, 250, 500 mg	250 mg 2–3 times/day (125 mg 2 times/day elderly) (max 2 g/day)	Contraindicated in depression, active liver disease, phaeochromocytoma, porphyria; caution in hepatic and renal impairment	Gastrointestinal effects, dry mouth, stomatitis, bradycardia, exacerbation of angina, postural hypotension, oedema, sedation, headache, dizziness, myalgia, arthralgia, nightmares, depression, hepatitis, jaundice, pancreatitis, haemolytic anaemia, bone marrow depression, hypersensitivity reactions, myocarditis, pericarditis, rashes
Moxonidine	Physiotens	Tablet	200, 400 mcg	200 mcg mane increasing to 400 mcg (max 600 mcg in 2 divided doses)	Contraindicated in conduction disorders, history of angio-oedema, bradycardia, severe heart failure, severe coronary artery disease, unstable angina, pregnancy and breast feeding; caution in severe hepatic or renal impairment	Dry mouth, headache, fatigue, dizziness, nausea, sleep disturbance, asthenia, vasodilatation

Drug	Trade name	Preparation	Strength	Doses used in hypertension (adult)	Comments	Side-effects
Alpha-adrenoceptor blocking drugs						
Doxazosin	Cardura	Tablet	1, 2 mg	1 mg/day initially, increasing to 2 mg and 4 mg/day prn (max 16 mg/day)	Contraindicated in urinary incontinence; caution in hepatic impairment	Postural hypotension, dizziness, vertigo, headache, fatigue, asthenia, oedema, somnolence, nausea, rhinitis
	Cardura XL	M/R tablet	4, 8 mg	Initiate 4mg/day, titrate to 8mg/day if required (max 8mg/day)		
Indoramin	Baratol	Tablet	25 mg	25 mg 2 times/day initially (max 300 mg in 2–3 divided doses)	Contraindicated in urinary incontinence and established heart failure; caution in hepatic and renal impairment	Sedation, dizziness, depression, failure of ejaculation, dry mouth, nasal congestion, extrapyramidal effects, weight gain
Prazosin	Hypovase	Tablet	1, 2, 5 mg	1 mg 2–3 times/day initially (max 20 mg/day)	Contraindicated in urinary incontinence and congested heart failure; reduce dose in hepatic and renal impairment; caution in pregnancy and breast feeding	Postural hypotension, drowsiness, weakness, dizziness, headache, lack of energy, nausea, palpitations, urinary frequency, incontinence, priapism
Terazosin	Hytrin	Tablet	1, 2, 5, 10 mg	1 mg nocte increasing to 2–10 mg/day (max 20 mg)	Contraindicated in urinary incontinence	Postural hypotension, dizziness, lack of energy, peripheral oedema, urinary frequency, priapism

Drug	Trade name	Preparation	Strength	Doses used in hypertension (adult)	Comments	Side-effects
Angiotensin-converting enzyme inhibitors						
Captopril	Capoten	Tablet	12.5, 25, 50 mg	12.5 mg 2 times daily (6.25 mg 2 times daily) increasing to 25 mg 2 times daily with diuretic, elderly (max 150 mg)	Contraindicated in renovascular disease, aortic stenosis, outflow tract obstruction, porphyria and pregnancy; caution in renal impairment	Renal impairment, persistent dry cough, angio-oedema, rash, pancreatitis, upper respiratory tract effects, gastrointestinal effects, liver function abnormalities, headache, dizziness, fatigue, malaise, taste disturbance, myalgia, arthralgia, tachycardia, serum sickness, weight loss, stomatitis, photosensitivity, flushing
Captopril + hydrochlorothiazide (co-zidocapt)	Capozide LS	Tablet	25 + 12.5 mg, 50 + 25 mg	1 tablet/day	For mild/moderate hypertension in patients controlled by the individual components in the same proportions	See also hydrochlorothiazide
	Capozide	Tablet		1 tablet/day		
Cilazapril	Vascace	Tablet	500 mcg, 1, 2.5, 5 mg	1 mg/day (500 mcg/day with diuretic, renal impairment, elderly), maintenance 1–2.5 mg/day (max 5 mg/day)	Contraindicated in renovascular disease, aortic stenosis, outflow tract obstruction, severe hepatic impairment and pregnancy; caution in renal impairment	Renal impairment, persistent dry cough, angio-oedema, rash, pancreatitis, upper respiratory tract effects, gastrointestinal effects, liver function abnormalities, headache, dizziness, fatigue, malaise, taste disturbance, myalgia, arthralgia, dyspnoea, bronchitis

Angiotensin-converting enzyme inhibitors

Drug	Trade name	Preparation	Strength	Doses used in hypertension (adult)	Comments	Side-effects
Enalapril	Innovace	Tablet	2.5, 5, 10, 20 mg	5 mg/day (2.5 mg/day with diuretic, renal impairment, elderly), maintenance 20 mg/day (max 40 mg/day)	Contraindicated in renovascular disease, aortic stenosis, outflow tract obstruction, porphyria and pregnancy; caution in renal and hepatic impairment	Renal impairment, persistent dry cough, angio-oedema, rash, pancreatitis, upper respiratory tract effects, gastrointestinal effects, liver function abnormalities, headache, dizziness, fatigue, malaise, taste disturbance, myalgia, arthralgia, palpitations, arrhythmias, chest pain, syncope, cerebrovascular accident, anorexia, stomatitis, dermatological effects, confusion, depression, nervousness, insomnia, impotence
Enalapril + hydrochloro-thiazide	Innozide	Tablet	20 + 12.5 mg	1 tablet/day	For mild/moderate hypertension in patients controlled by the individual components in the same proportions	See also hydrochlorothiazide
Fosinopril	Staril	Tablet	10, 20 mg	10 mg/day (less with diuretic), maintenance 10–40 mg/day (max 40 mg/day)	Contraindicated in renovascular disease, aortic stenosis, outflow tract obstruction, severe hepatic impairment, porphyria and pregnancy; caution in renal impairment	Renal impairment, persistent dry cough, angio-oedema, rash, pancreatitis, upper respiratory tract effects, gastrointestinal effects, liver function abnormalities, headache, dizziness, fatigue, malaise, taste disturbance, myalgia, arthralgia, chest pain, musculoskeletal pain

Drug	Trade name	Preparation	Strength	Doses used in hypertension (adult)	Comments	Side-effects
Angiotensin-converting enzyme inhibitors						
Imidapril	Tanatril	Tablet	5, 10, 20 mg	5 mg/day (2.5 mg/day with diuretic, heart failure, cerebrovascular disease, angina, renal or hepatic impairment, elderly); maintenance 10 mg/day (max 20 mg/day)	Contraindicated in renovascular disease, aortic stenosis, outflow tract obstruction and pregnancy; caution in renal and hepatic impairment	Renal impairment, persistent dry cough, angio-oedema, rash, pancreatitis, upper respiratory tract effects, gastrointestinal effects, liver function abnormalities, headache, dizziness, fatigue, malaise, taste disturbance, myalgia, arthralgia, dry mouth, glossitis, abdominal pain, bronchitis, sleep disturbances, depression, confusion, blurred vision, tinnitus, impotence
Lisinopril	Carace	Tablet	2.5, 5, 10, 20 mg	2.5 mg/day, maintenance 10–20 mg/day (max 40 mg/day)	Contraindicated in renovascular disease, aortic stenosis, outflow tract obstruction and pregnancy; caution in renal impairment	Renal impairment, persistent dry cough, angio-oedema, rash, pancreatitis, upper respiratory tract effects, gastrointestinal effects, liver function abnormalities, headache, dizziness, fatigue, malaise, taste disturbance, myalgia, tachycardia, cerebrovascular accident, myocardial infarction, dry mouth, confusion, mood changes, asthenia, sweating, impotence
	Zestril	Tablet	2.5, 5, 10, 20 mg			
Lisinopril + hydrochloro-thiazide	Carace Plus	Tablet	10 + 12.5 mg, 20 + 12.5 mg	1 tablet/day	For mild/moderate hypertension in patients controlled by the individual components in the same proportions	See also hydrochlorothiazide
	Zestoretic	Tablet	10 + 12.5 mg, 20 + 12.5 mg	1 tablet/day		

Drug	Trade name	Preparation	Strength	Doses used in hypertension (adult)	Comments	Side-effects
Angiotensin-converting enzyme inhibitors						
Moexipril	Perdix	Tablet	7.5, 15 mg	7.5 mg/day (3.75 mg/day with diuretic, renal or hepatic impairment, elderly), maintenance 15–30 mg/day (max 30 mg/day)	Contraindicated in renovascular disease, aortic stenosis, outflow tract obstruction and pregnancy; caution in renal and hepatic impairment	Renal impairment, persistent dry cough, angio-oedema, rash, pancreatitis, upper respiratory tract effects, gastrointestinal effects, liver function abnormalities, headache, dizziness, fatigue, malaise, taste disturbance, myalgia, tachycardia, arrhythmias, angina, chest pain, syncope, cerebrovascular accident, myocardial infarction, appetite and weight changes, dry mouth, photosensitivity, flushing, nervousness, mood changes, anxiety, drowsiness sleep disturbance
Perindopril	Coversyl	Tablet	2, 4 mg	2 mg/day (less with diuretic), maintenance 4 mg/day (max 8 mg/day)	Contraindicated in renovascular disease, aortic stenosis, outflow tract obstruction and pregnancy; caution in renal and hepatic impairment	Renal impairment, persistent dry cough, angio-oedema, rash, pancreatitis, upper respiratory tract effects, gastrointestinal effects, liver function abnormalities, headache, dizziness, fatigue, malaise, taste disturbance, myalgia, tachycardia, asthenia, flushing, mood and sleep disturbances

Drug	Trade name	Preparation	Strength	Doses used in hypertension (adult)	Comments	Side-effects
Angiotensin-converting enzyme inhibitors						
Quinapril	Accupro	Tablet	5, 10, 20, 40 mg	10 mg/day (2.5 mg with diuretic, renal impairment, elderly). maintenance 20–40 mg/day (max 80 mg/day)	Contraindicated in renovascular disease, aortic stenosis, outflow tract obstruction and pregnancy; caution in renal and hepatic impairment	Renal impairment, persistent dry cough, angio-oedema, rash, pancreatitis, upper respiratory tract effects, gastrointestinal effects, liver function abnormalities, headache, dizziness, fatigue, malaise, taste disturbance, myalgia, tachycardia, asthenia, chest pain, oedema, flatulence, nervousness, insomnia, blurred vision, impotence, back pain, myalgia
Quinapril + hydrochloro-thiazide	Accuretic	Tablet	10 + 12.5 mg	1 tablet/day	For mild/moderate hypertension in patients controlled by the individual components in the same proportions	See also hydrochlorothiazide
Ramipril	Tritace	Tablet	1.25, 2.5, 5, 10 mg	1.25 mg/day (less with diuretic). maintenance 2.5–5 mg/day (max 10 mg/day)	Contraindicated in renovascular disease, aortic stenosis, outflow tract obstruction and pregnancy; caution in renal and hepatic impairment	Renal impairment, persistent dry cough, angio-oedema, rash, pancreatitis, upper respiratory tract effects, gastrointestinal effects, liver function abnormalities, headache, dizziness, fatigue, malaise, taste disturbance, myalgia, tachycardia, arrhythmias, angina, chest pain, myocardial infarction, loss of appetite, dry mouth, dermatological effects, confusion, nervousness, depression, anxiety, impotence, bronchitis, muscle cramps

Drug	Trade name	Preparation	Strength	Doses used in hypertension (adult)	Comments	Side-effects
Angiotensin-converting enzyme inhibitors						
Ramipril + felodipine	Triapin Mite	Tablet	2.5 + 2.5 mg	1 tablet/day	For hypertension in patients controlled by the individual components in the same proportions	See also felodipine
	Triapin	Tablet	5 + 5 mg	1 tablet/day		
Trandolapril	Gopten	Capsule	1, 2 mg	500 mcg/day (less with diuretic), maintenance 1–2 mg/day (max 4 mg/day)	Contraindicated in renovascular disease, aortic stenosis, outflow tract obstruction and pregnancy; caution in renal and hepatic impairment	Renal impairment, persistent dry cough, angio-oedema, rash, pancreatitis, upper respiratory tract effects, gastrointestinal effects, liver function abnormalities, headache, dizziness, fatigue, malaise, taste disturbance, myalgia, tachycardia, arrhythmias, angina, chest pain, cerebral haemorrhage, myocardial infarction, dry mouth, dermatological effects, asthenia, alopecia, dyspnoea, bronchitis
	Odrik	Capsule	500 mcg, 1, 2 mg			
Trandolapril + verapamil	Tarka	Capsule	1 + 180, 2 + 180, 2 + 240, 4 + 240 mg	1 capsule/day	For hypertension in patients controlled by the individual components in the same proportions	See also verapamil

Drug	Trade name	Preparation	Strength	Doses used in hypertension (adult)	Comments	Side-effects
Angiotensin II receptor antagonists						
Candesartan	Amias	Tablet	4, 8, 16, 32 mg	4 mg/day (2 mg in hepatic and renal impairment), maintenance 8 mg (max 16 mg)	Contraindicated in pregnancy and breast feeding; caution in aortic or mitral valve stenosis, obstructive hypertrophic cardiomyopathy, renal and hepatic impairment	Symptomatic hypotension, hyperkalaemia, upper respiratory tract symptoms, abdominal pain, back pain, arthralgia, myalgia, nausea, headache, dizziness, peripheral oedema, rash
Eprosartan	Teveten	Tablet	400, 600 mg	600 mg/day (300 mg/day >75 years, hepatic and renal impairment), maintenance 800 mg/day	Contraindicated in pregnancy and breast feeding; caution in aortic or mitral valve stenosis, obstructive hypertrophic cardiomyopathy, renal and hepatic impairment	Symptomatic hypotension, hyperkalaemia, flatulence, dizziness, arthralgia, rhinitis, hypertriglyceridaemia
Irbesartan	Aprovel	Tablet	75, 150, 300 mg	150 mg/day (75 mg/day >75 years), maintenance 300 mg/day	Contraindicated in pregnancy and breast feeding; caution in aortic or mitral valve stenosis, obstructive hypertrophic cardiomyopathy, renal and hepatic impairment	Symptomatic hypotension, hyperkalaemia, diarrhoea, dyspepsia, flushing, tachycardia, dizziness, asthenia, myalgia, rash, urticaria

Angiotensin II receptor antagonists

Drug	Trade name	Preparation	Strength	Doses used in hypertension (adult)	Comments	Side-effects
Ibesartan + hydrochloro-thiazide	CoAprovel	Tablet	150 + 12.5, 300 + 12.5 mg	1 tablet/day	For hypertension in patients controlled by the individual components in the same proportions	See also hydrochlorothiazide
Losartan	Cozaar	Tablet	25, 50, 100 mg	50 mg/day (25 mg/day >75 years, severe renal impairment) (max 100 mg/day)	Contraindicated in pregnancy and breast feeding; caution in aortic or mitral valve stenosis, obstructive hypertrophic cardiomyopathy, renal and hepatic impairment	Symptomatic hypotension, hyperkalaemia, diarrhoea, dizziness, taste disturbance, cough, myalgia, migraine, urticaria, pruritus, rash
Losartan + hydrochloro-thiazide	Cozaar Comp	Tablet	50 + 12.5, 100 + 25 mg	1 tablet/day	For hypertension in patients controlled by the individual components in the same proportions	See also hydrochlorothiazide
Telmisartan	Micardis	Tablet	20, 40, 80 mg	40 mg/day (max 80 mg/day)	Contraindicated in biliary obstruction, gastric or duodenal ulceration, pregnancy and breast feeding; caution in aortic or mitral valve stenosis, obstructive hypertrophic cardiomyopathy, renal and hepatic impairment	Symptomatic hypotension, hyperkalaemia, gastrointestinal effects, pharyngitis, back pain, myalgia

Drug	Trade name	Preparation	Strength	Doses used in hypertension (adult)	Comments	Side-effects
Angiotensin II receptor antagonists						
Valsartan	Diovan	Caplet	40, 80, 160 mg	80 mg/day (40 mg/day >75 years, renal and hepatic impairment) (max 160 mg/day)	Contraindicated in biliary obstruction, cirrhosis, pregnancy and breast feeding; caution in aortic or mitral valve stenosis, obstructive hypertrophic cardiomyopathy, renal and hepatic impairment	Symptomatic hypotension, hyperkalaemia, fatigue
Calcium channel blockers						
Amlodipine	Istin	Tablet	5, 10 mg	5 mg/day (max 10 mg/day)	Contraindicated in cardiogenic shock, unstable angina, aortic stenosis, pregnancy and breast feeding; caution in renal and hepatic impairment	Headache, oedema, fatigue, nausea, flushing, dizziness, gum hyperplasia, rashes
Diltiazem	Adizem-SR	M/R capsule	90, 120, 180 mg	120 mg 2 times/day (max 180 mg 2 times/day)	Contraindicated in severe bradycardia, second or third degree atrioventricular block, sick sinus syndrome, pregnancy and breast feeding; reduce dose in hepatic or renal failure or significantly impaired left ventricular function, bradycardia, first degree atrioventricular block or prolonged PR interval; patients should be maintained on the same brand because of	Bradycardia, sino-atrial block, atrioventricular block, palpitations, dizziness, symptomatic hypotension, malaise, asthenia, headache, hot flushes, gastrointestinal effects, constipation, oedema
	Adizem-XL	M/R tablet	120 mg			
		M/R tablet	120, 180, 240, 300 mg	240 mg/day (120 mg/day elderly, renal and hepatic impairment) (max 300 mg/day)		

Drug	Trade name	Preparation	Strength	Doses used in hypertension (adult)	Comments	Side-effects
Calcium channel blockers						
Diltiazem cont...	Dilzem SR	M/R capsule	60, 90, 120 mg	90 mg 2 times/day (60 mg 2 times/day elderly) (max 180 mg 2 times/day	variations in clinical effect; all formulations should be swallowed whole; do not use with beta-adrenoceptor blocking drugs	
	Dilzem XL	M/R capsule	120, 180, 240 mg	180 mg/day (120 mg/day elderly, renal and hepatic impairment) (max 360 mg/day)		
	Tildiem LA	M/R capsule	200, 300 mg	200 mg/day, maintenance 300–400 mg/day (max 500 mg/day, elderly, renal and hepatic impairment 300 mg/day)		
	Tildiem Retard	M/R tablet	90, 120 mg	90–120 mg 2 times/day (120 mg/day elderly, hepatic or renal impairment), (max 360 mg/day in divided doses)		

Drug	Trade name	Preparation	Strength	Doses used in hypertension (adult)	Comments	Side-effects
Calcium channel blockers						
Felodipine	Plendil	Tablet	2.5, 5, 10 mg	5 mg mane (2.5 mg mane elderly). maintenance 5–10 mg mane (max 20 mg mane)	Contraindicated in unstable angina, uncontrolled heart failure, aortic stenosis, within 1 month of myocardial infarction and pregnancy; caution in renal and hepatic impairment; swallow whole	Flushing, headache, palpitations, dizziness, fatigue, gravitational oedema
Isradipine	Prescal	Tablet	2.5, 5 mg	2.5 mg 2 times/day (25 mg 2 times/day elderly, hepatic or renal impairment); maintenance 2.5–10 mg/day (max 10 mg 2 times/day) CR – dose once daily	Contraindicated in tight aortic stenosis, sick sinus syndrome and pregnancy; caution in renal and hepatic impairment	Headache, flushing, dizziness, tachycardia, palpitations, localized peripheral oedema
Lacidipine	Motens	Tablet	2, 4 mg	2 mg mane, maintenance 4 mg mane (max 6 mg mane)	Contraindicated in aortic stenosis, within 1 month of myocardial infarction, pregnancy and breast feeding; caution in renal and hepatic impairment	Headache, flushing, oedema, dizziness, palpitations
Lercanidipine	Zanidip	Tablet	10, 20 mg	10 mg/day (max 20 mg/day; max may be 40 mg in the USA)	Contraindicated in aortic stenosis, unstable angina, uncontrolled heart failure, within 1 month of myocardial infarction and pregnancy; caution in renal and hepatic impairment, left ventricular dysfunction, sick sinus syndrome; take before food	Flushing, peripheral oedema, palpitations, tachycardia, headache, dizziness, asthenia

Drug	Trade name	Preparation	Strength	Doses used in hypertension (adult)	Comments	Side-effects
Calcium channel blockers						
Nicardipine	Cardene	Capsule	10, 20 mg	20 mg 3 times/day, maintenance 60–120 mg/day	Contraindicated in cardiogenic shock, aortic stenosis, unstable angina, within 1 month of myocardial infarction. Caution in pregnancy and breast feeding; caution in congestive heart failure, impaired left ventricular function, renal and hepatic impairment; M/R formulation should be swallowed whole	Dizziness, headache, peripheral oedema, flushing, palpitations, nausea
	Cardene SR	M/R capsule	30, 45 mg	30 mg 2 times/day, maintenance 30–60 mg 2 times/day		
Nifedipine	Adalat LA	M/R tablet	20, 30, 60 mg	20 mg/day initially	Contraindicated in cardiogenic shock, advanced aortic stenosis, unstable angina, within 1 month of myocardial infarction, porphyria; caution in pregnancy and breast feeding; congestive heart failure, impaired left ventricular function, renal and hepatic impairment; patients should be maintained on the same brand because of variations in clinical effect; all formulations should be swallowed whole	Headache, flushing, dizziness, lethargy, tachycardia, palpitations, gravitational oedema, rash, pruritus, urticaria, nausea, constipation, visual disturbances, gum hyperplasia, paraesthesia, impotence, depression
	Adalat Retard	M/R tablet	10, 20 mg	10 mg 2 times/day (max 40 mg 2 times/day)		
	Adipine MR	M/R tablet	10, 20 mg	10 mg 2 times/day (max 40 mg 2 times/day)		
	Coracten SR	M/R capsule	10, 20 mg	20 mg 2 times/day, maintenance 10–40 mg 2 times/day		
	Coracten XL	M/R capsule	30, 60 mg	30 mg/day (max 90 mg/day)		

Drug	Trade name	Preparation	Strength	Doses used in hypertension (adult)	Comments	Side-effects
Calcium channel blockers						
Nifedipine cont...	Fortipine LA 40	M/R tablet	40 mg	40 mg/day (max 80 mg/day)	Contraindicated in cardiogenic shock, aortic stenosis, unstable angina, within 1 month of myocardial infarction, hepatic impairment, pregnancy and breast feeding; caution in renal impairment: swallow whole	Gravitational oedema, headache, flushing, tachycardia, palpitations, dizziness, asthenia, gastrointestinal effects
Nisoldipine	Syscor MR	M/R tablet	10, 20, 30, 40 mg	10 mg daily (max 40 mg daily)		
Verapamil	Cordilox	Tablet	40, 80, 120, 160 mg	240–480 mg/day in 2–3 divided doses	Contraindicated in bradycardia, second or third degree atrioventricular block, sick sinus syndrome, cardiogenic shock, sino-atrial block, impaired left ventricular function, porphyria; caution in first degree atrioventricular block, acute phase of myocardial infarction, hepatic impairment, pregnancy and breast feeding; do not use with beta-adrenoceptor blocking drugs; M/R formulations should be swallowed whole	Constipation, nausea, vomiting, flushing, headache, dizziness, fatigue, ankle oedema
	Securon	Tablet	40, 120 mg	120 mg/day, maintenance		
	Half Securon SR	M/R tablet	120 mg			
	Securon SR	M/R tablet	240 mg	240 mg/day (max 480 mg/day)		
	Univer	M/R capsule	120, 180, 240 mg	240 mg/day (max 480 mg/day)		

Appendix 2 – Useful Addresses and Websites

For the physician
Societies

American College of Cardiology
Address: Heart House, 9111 Old Georgetown Road, Bethesda
MD 20814-1699, USA
Tel.: (800) 253 4636, ext. 694
Fax: (301) 897 9745
Website: http://www.acc.org/

American Diabetes Association
Address: (Attn: National Call Center), 1701 North Beauregard
Street, Alexandria, VA 22311, USA
Tel.: 800 342 2383
Website: http://www.diabetes.org

American Heart Association
Address: One North Franklin, Chicago, IL 60606-3421, USA
Tel.: 312 422 3000
Website: http://www.aha.org

American Society of Hypertension
Address: 148 Madison Avenue, New York, NY 10016, USA
Tel.: 212 696 9099
Fax: 212 696 0711
E-mail: ash@ash-us.org
Website: http://www.ash-us.org/

American Stroke Association
Address: National Center, 7272 Greenville Avenue, Dallas
TX 75231, USA
Tel.: 1 800 242 8721
Website: http://www.strokeassociation.org

Blood Pressure Association
Address: 60 Cranmer Terrace, London SW17 0QS, UK
Website: http://www.bpassoc.org.uk
Tel.: +44 (0)20 8772 4994
Fax: +44 (0)20 8772 4999

British Cardiac Society
Address: 9 Fitzroy Square, London W1T 5HW, UK
Tel.:+44 20 7383 3887
Fax: +44 20 7388 0903
Website: http://www.bcs.com

British Hypertension Society
Address: Blood Pressure Unit, Department of Physiological
Medicine, St George's Hospital Medical School, Cranmer Terrace,
London SW17 ORE, UK
Tel.: +44 20 8725 3412
Fax: +44 20 8725 2959
E-mail: bhsis@sghms.ac.uk
Website: http://www.hyp.ac.uk/bhs

European Atherosclerosis Society
Address: Secretary, Dr. Sebastiano Calandra, Sezione di Patologia
Generale, Dipartimento di Scienze Biomediche, Universita di
Modena e Reggio Emilia, Via Campi 287, I-41100 Modena, Italy
Fax: +39 059 2055 426
Website://www.elsevier.com/inca/homepage/sab/eas/menu.htm

European Society of Cardiology
Address: The European Heart House, 2035 Route des Colles
B.P. 179 – Les Templiers, FR-06903 Sophia Antipolis, France
E-mail: webmaster@escardio.org
Website: http://www.escardio.org

European Society of Hypertension
Address: Inst. Clinical Exp. Medicine, Dept of Preventive
Cardiology. Videnska 1958/9. 140 21 Prague 4. Czech Republic
Tel.: +1 613 761 4785
Fax: +1 613 761 5309
Website: http://www.eshonline.org

Primary Care Diabetes UK
Address: 10 Parkway, London NW1 7AA, UK
Tel.: +44 20 7424 1000
Fax: +44 20 7424 1001
E-mail: info@diabetes.org.uk
Website: http://www.diabetes.org.uk/home.htm

Journals

Chest
Journal of the American College of Chest Physicians
http://www.chestjournal.org/

Heart Journal
http://heart.bmjjournals.com/

Stroke
Journal of the American Heart Association
http://stroke.ahajournals.org/

For the patient
Societies

American Diabetes Association
(see above)

British Heart Foundation
14 Fitzhardinge Street, London W1H 6DH, UK
Tel.: +44 20 7935 0185
Fax: +44 20 7486 5820
E-mail: internet@bhf.org.uk
Website: http://www.bhf.org.uk

Primary Care Diabetes UK
(see above)

Index

As hypertension is the subject of this book, all index entries refer to hypertension unless otherwise indicated.

Page numbers followed by 'f' indicate figures: page numbers followed by 't' indicate tables.

This index is in letter-by-letter order, whereby spaces and hyphens in main entries are excluded from the alphabetization process.

Cross references between proprietary drug names and generic names are assumed and not given.